From Oncology Nursing to
Coping with Breast Cancer

From Oncology Nursing to Coping with Breast Cancer

My journey there and back

KATE HAYWARD

Radcliffe Publishing
Oxford • New York

Radcliffe Publishing Ltd
18 Marcham Road
Abingdon
Oxon OX14 1AA
United Kingdom

www.radcliffe-oxford.com
Electronic catalogue and worldwide online ordering facility.

British Library Cataloguing in Publication Data

A catalogue record for this book is available from the British Library.

ISBN-13: 978 184619 273 9

The books in the Patient Narratives series provide first-hand accounts of experiences of illness. Sometimes gruelling, sometimes uplifting, each personal description vividly illustrates the highs and lows of being a patient, where treatment can be good or bad, unsuccessful or successful, and the insights are invaluable. Visit www.radcliffe-oxford.com/patientnarratives

Typeset by Pindar NZ (Egan Reid), Auckland, New Zealand
Printed and bound by TJI Digital, Padstow, Cornwall, UK

This book is dedicated to three very important men who I couldn't have lived without; my lovely husband Phil Hayward, my surgeon Mr Philip Turton MBChB, FRCS Ed, FRCE (Gen Surg), MD (Hons) and Dr Timothy J Perren MD, FRCP Consultant Medical Oncologist. I can't thank you enough for helping me.

Preface

'Above all what matters is not to lose the joy of living in the fear of dying.'[1]

Many healthcare professionals that I've encountered refer to a patient's cancer journey; indeed I had an article published in 2004, describing a patient's journey through biological therapy.[2] This particular case history described my involvement with a medical doctor's experience of renal cell carcinoma and self-administration of immunotherapy. He was very keen to share his experience to educate and inform other health professionals and I now find myself in a similar situation.

In March 2006, I 'journeyed' from nurse to patient when diagnosed with grade 3-breast cancer. Of course, I've experienced various health problems before this time, but I've never spent a night in hospital, unlike members of my family who've experienced serious illness and hospitalisation on several occasions. Consequently I've always regarded myself in the caring role amongst family members and over the years I've used my nursing knowledge and skills to help them deal with both the physical and psychological issues of their various disease processes. However, being diagnosed with breast cancer has now changed me from nurse and carer into a vulnerable ill person with doubts and fears for my future. To restore some sense of purpose while on sick leave and help me to get through each treatment stage, I decided to keep a daily journal of my experience. I've been as honest as I can but I want some aspects of the traumatic last two years or so to remain between my husband Phil and myself.

Kate Hayward
May 2008

Author's note

Cookridge Hospital has since merged with St James's in the new Bexley Wing 'state of the art' St James's Institute of Oncology. Information on many issues, such as cancer types, clinical trials and research can be obtained at www.cancerresearchuk.org.

Kate Hayward
May 2008

Kate's story

When I was a little girl, my parents Joan and Harold (affectionately called Joaney and Pop by me) bought me a nurses outfit for Christmas, and I loved bandaging the dog and giving 'Dolly Mixture' sweets as tablets to my brother Steve. I decided that I wanted to be a nurse from the first time I put on the white cap, apron and cuffs with their bright red crosses. I had a very happy childhood, living in a small village next to the primary school I attended. In fact I couldn't wait until I was old enough to go and used to sneak through our back garden into the classes with Judy our dog. Joaney had to come and find me in whichever classroom I fancied that particular day. None of the teachers minded though and didn't want to curb my enthusiasm for learning. I couldn't understand why other children were crying on my first official day there, as I was so happy!

My parents told me recently that I started using my 'nursing skills' at every opportunity when someone fell over in the playground. Apparently I asked the headmaster to move the first aid kit to a lower shelf, as I couldn't reach it to get dressings for cuts and grazes. Moving to the grammar school wasn't quite as enjoyable as I've always hated written examinations and I struggled at times with the science subjects I'd chosen. However my form teacher wrote in the end of year report that I was a 'tonic' in his daily life and that really pleased me as I thought it was preferable to help people feel better than be purely academic.

My decision to be a nurse never wavered through secondary school and luckily I achieved good enough 'O' level results to be accepted at St James's University Hospital in Leeds to train as a State Registered Nurse. It was there at our entrance interviews in 1975 that I met Wilma, who's been a fantastic friend and support to me throughout my life since then. At the start of our training we shared the very basic nurse's home accommodation and over the last thirty years we've been on holiday together, I've stayed at her house when working a late and early shift to save extra travelling and she came to stay with me when I moved to the Midlands during my first marriage. We've laughed and cried together during good and bad times and she's one of only two of my old friends who've been to both my weddings!

My nursing career has been quite varied, with experience in intensive care, spinal injuries, trauma and orthopaedics, coronary care, infectious diseases in babies up to one-year-old and bone marrow transplantation (BMT). It was during my time on the BMT unit that I attended a nursing conference and one of the topics was breast cancer when the statistics were approximately 1:12 women. I clearly remember counting the row of women I was sitting with and there were 12 of us in the row. As I was thinking, 'that means one of us could get it' the woman sitting next to me leaned over and said 'don't worry, it's me as I've had it' and she got up to deliver the lecture as I breathed a sigh of relief. Of course now the odds have been reduced to 1:9 women and I'm one of the 8,000 women below 50 years of age at diagnosis in the UK.[3]

Luckily, over my nursing career I've made lots of friends from the medical and nursing profession and many of them have been a huge support to me through the ups and downs of my life. Since I was diagnosed with breast cancer and living through the trauma of the past 14 months or so, I've needed them more than ever.

'MILLS & BOON STUFF'

I married my school sweetheart during the third year of training but sadly we grew apart. We separated in 1989 and I was on my own for a couple of years. Then, while working in oncology I met my second husband, Phil. I feel blessed to have had such a happy second marriage as Phil's my soul mate and the absolute love of my life.

I know there are lots of 'hospital romance' stories, indeed many of my friends are doctors married to other doctors or nurses. However, I married Phil after meeting him as a patient. Initially I was struck by his bravery at being recalled by the hospital from the airport as he was about to go on holiday. I was working in clinic with Professor Peter Selby who asked me to stay for the consultation with Phil. He told him that he needed treatment with high-dose chemotherapy and that, as he has no siblings, a bone marrow autotransplant. This needed to be done as a matter of urgency to arrest the recurrence of his Hodgkin's lymphoma that had plagued him since his twenties. I remember feeling great empathy towards him at that point and wished him well with his treatment, as that would be undertaken by the haematologists.

Before his admission for the transplant I met him as an out-patient to administer some chemotherapy, and as he has fair, freckly skin (notoriously difficult to cannulate) I spent some time stroking his hand to encourage the blood flow to his veins. He asked me 'What does your husband think to you doing a job like this?' and I remember feeling embarrassed and muttering something like 'err he's not around anymore'. This comment stuck in Phil's mind and at the time I didn't know that he was also having problems in his marriage.

As time went on, I rang the ward to enquire about his progress and was pleased to hear he was doing well. Then, weeks later, he rang me to see if he could come and ask me some questions about his recovery post-transplant. Of course I agreed as I wanted to help him as I would with any patient. He arrived in my office looking extremely handsome and tanned as he'd just returned from holiday. He had several worries about his stamina and progress which we talked about but he also told me that he'd separated from his wife. It was then that he asked me 'How do we start again after being in a long relationship?' I told him that I never refused an offer from my friends and would 'go to the opening of curtains!!' rather than being on my own. He thought his illness would be a barrier to meeting new people, but I remember saying that if we'd met in a pub I'd have no idea of what he'd been through and tried to reassure him that there was life after a break-up.

It took him a while to pluck up courage, but then he rang to ask me out for dinner and I had very mixed feelings. On the one hand I reasoned that although a patient, I'd only ever seen him fully dressed, but equally the ethical dilemma of 'dating' reared its head. Equally I didn't want to dismiss him and deflate his confidence. In the end I turned to Prof Selby for advice and he told me 'he's a lovely chap, you're both single, go for it!' There was no denying the chemistry between us at the last meeting and with Peter's blessing I agreed to meet him on 10th December 1991 for a meal. A lasting joke between us from that night is that I told him 'I don't eat puddings thank you' when he asked if I wanted dessert, as I didn't want to appear greedy. Now he knows that was an absolute lie as I pick my dessert before I look at the main course on a menu! I like to think we fell a little bit in love that night but I was absolutely sure by Christmas. We remained a happy, reasonably carefree couple until March 1992.

Phil broke his leg on a skiing trip with a friend and I met him from the plane from Austria as he was transferred to St James's. I was concerned that he was feverish and looked unwell and was devastated when Peter diagnosed another relapse of the Hodgkin's lymphoma. This was just a year after the autotransplant and he had to undergo more chemotherapy. That's when I moved in with him to help him through the treatment and stop him breaking his other leg while getting used to the crutches! We were very relieved when further chemotherapy treatment was successful. So cancer has always been a threat to us and poor Peter's been our very own 'agony uncle' for advice and helping us to sort out our health issues. Not only has he treated Phil but he also helped me to get treatment for a benign breast lump in the summer of 1992 and referred us, after much deliberation, for in vitro fertilisation (IVF) just after we got married in 1995. In fact, Peter once told me my life was like a 'soap opera'.

At times I've felt that fate has played a huge hand in my life, leading to both good and bad conclusions. So when I was undergoing the IVF treatment I used to bargain with God in my mind that I didn't want to have a child at the expense of Phil ever being ill again, as I couldn't live happily without him. I subsequently had two successful pregnancies but sadly miscarried both times. We've since learnt to be content with one another but that means our very close relationship constantly feels under threat and vulnerable to forces beyond our control.

FROM ONCOLOGY NURSE TO PATIENT

I have worked as a Clinical Nurse Specialist [CNS] in the Oncology Department at St James's Hospital in Leeds, since February 1990. In 1998 my role diversified from cytotoxic chemotherapy delivery to biological therapy for renal cell carcinoma and malignant melanoma patients. The majority of these treatments are administered in the outpatient setting involving self-injection or utilising support from the primary care teams. Consequently, my role as CNS is to provide a nurse-led service for education, monitoring, support and liaison with patients, relatives, and hospital and primary care teams.[4] Prior to this, I was instrumental in establishing the chemotherapy service and intravenous therapy nursing team (IV team), for both ward and outpatients. I greatly enjoyed the practical elements of the post and the close relationships developed with my patients and their relatives throughout their treatment. I don't think I'm the perfect nurse but I've endeavoured to use evidence-based practice to support, educate and treat patients along with empathy and compassion. Now I'm a patient myself, I've found it quite difficult at times to stop thinking as a nurse and 'behave' like a patient. So, I'm sure I've not been the 'perfect' patient either!

HOW IT ALL STARTED

The first entry in my journal was on 1st March 2006, but my story should really have started during the Christmas holidays in 2005 when I first felt an obvious lump in the lower, outer area of my left breast, as I was in the bath. I remember thinking that it was probably due to hormones or a similar benign lump to one I'd had treated with evening primrose oil capsules. I chose to monitor changes in my left breast myself, not wishing to be thought overly cautious by my GP and probably also suffering from a certain amount of denial. I couldn't believe that it could be malignant, as this was Christmas and I didn't want bad things to happen at Christmas. I didn't want to spoil our family time. So I checked my chest area in the mirror and couldn't see any puckering of the skin or peau d'orange skin.[5] However, I didn't lift my arm up until after the diagnosis and when I did this the dimpling was obvious.

In retrospect, I had been aware of a difference since the previous summer when I had had to buy larger bras as the cup-size of both breasts had increased, but more so on the left. It's well recognised that some degree of asymmetry is common and usually it will be the left breast that is slightly larger.[6] So I largely ignored it and must admit I was quite pleased at that particular change as, for the first time in my life, I had a decent cleavage! Also, despite a healthy diet and reasonable amount of exercise, being in my late forties I assumed the changes were due to general weight gain.

During January and February I kept feeling the area and thinking I should get it checked out for peace of mind, as it wasn't going away on its own. I decided to contact my GP for a check after returning from a planned long weekend in the North Yorkshire moors with Phil and our friends Mark and Keri. Ironically, on holiday I was reading Gloria Hunniford's book, *Next to You*,[7] describing her daughter's experience of breast cancer, when I rolled over on the bed and became aware of a tugging sensation underneath the breast. The lump was definitely larger and felt quite solid. There was now no doubt in my mind about the necessity of a GP appointment and I decided to arrange one as soon as we returned home. I think I knew at that moment that it was breast cancer but of course hoped I was wrong.

Phil was completely unaware of any problem as I had decided to wait until I had confirmation of whether the lump was benign or malignant before I told him. A few weeks earlier he'd noticed a prominent vein on my chest and commented on it. I told him it was probably my skin thinning due to getting older.

Unfortunately the car broke down as we set off home from the holiday and he probably wondered why I was so tetchy about the delay. I nearly told him about my worries but decided it would be difficult for him to deal with the breakdown mechanic after such news. As events turned out it was just two days later, at the Breast Unit at St James's, that I knew our lives were to change in 2006.

I rang the GP surgery as soon as we arrived home and booked the next available appointment, which turned out to be a whole week later. Naturally I was concerned at having to wait but rationalised I'd probably waited too long anyway, so another few days wouldn't really matter. So I returned to work on Tuesday

28th February and tried to concentrate on my patients' worries rather than my own. As usual, I went to the Parkway Hotel leisure centre after work for my nightly swim. This always relaxes me for the evening and helps to keep my bad back in better shape. I enjoyed the time in the steam room more than the swim but any relaxation I'd achieved was quickly dispelled when I was showering. Overnight, it seemed the lump was larger still, harder and also I could feel firm strands of tissue connected to my ribcage (I later found out these were the Coopers ligaments that I could feel). These are the ligaments that help to support the breast against the chest and can stretch with obesity, age and prolonged breast-feeding. These ligaments can shrink when affected by malignancy and this causes the skin to pucker.[8] By now there was little doubt in my mind that this was a malignant lump. I decided to bypass waiting for the GP appointment and the next morning went to the Breast Unit at St James's and explained my findings to Belinda, one of the breast care nurses whom I've known for many years. In this respect, I was very lucky to get investigations so quickly as I was on the hospital site and able to call upon healthcare colleagues to see me in the afternoon.

March 2006–May 2007
My breast cancer journal

CONFIRMATION OF MALIGNANCY

1 MARCH 2006

Belinda was brilliant and organised a mammogram and ultrasound for later that day. It was very difficult trying to maintain normality in the office I share with nursing friends and they were aware that 'something was going on', as I was quite subdued. I guessed the news wasn't good when the mammogram and ultrasound took a while to perform and just by observing the radiographer's expression, but I wasn't prepared for the news that I also had a problem with calcification in the right breast, which would also need a biopsy. So I walked back to the office with the knowledge that the left breast lump was very likely malignant and the right side would also need investigation. As soon as I saw my friends I burst into tears and explained what I knew. Gill's the Lymphoma Clinical Nurse Specialist but her previous post had been in breast care and Catherine was leader of the IV team so I was in very good hands for advice and support. They decided the best course of action was to come home with me and open some wine! This was how Phil found us later that evening as he returned home slightly earlier than usual, before Gill and Catherine had left. He looked a bit annoyed with us and was obviously puzzled why we were at home drinking wine. So my carefully planned explanation was blurted out when they left us alone.

I explained about having the mammogram and ultrasound. Poor Phil nearly fainted. I told him to be prepared for the worst outcome of disease in both breasts and that I'd know more after seeing the surgeon the next day. I felt so guilty for causing him such distress and he said how unfair he felt life was, as he thought we'd had our share of bad luck with his own health problems and the failed in vitro fertilisation (IVF) treatment at the start of our marriage.

2 MARCH 2006

I went to the Breast Unit and met one of the surgeons, Phil Turton, who was 99% certain of breast cancer after examining me. The lump I could feel was malignant but he also told me of other suspicious areas that I was unaware of. I wasn't shocked by the diagnosis as I was expecting it, but I did swear as I felt I had to make some response. To be honest it was almost a relief as I'd had a 'bad' feeling for some months that I was going to have to deal with bad news and I was glad it was me and not Phil or anyone else in my family. Also I had the incidence statistics buzzing through my mind and couldn't help thinking that I'd joined one of the 40,000 plus other women diagnosed each year. In 2003 there were 44,100 new cases diagnosed in the UK.[9]

It felt weird having to strip off while I was officially at work, so I tried to visualise being on the beach sunbathing topless! I was really glad to have Gill with me for a second pair of ears as I had agreed with Phil that he'd go to work and wait for me to ring him. Phil Turton did cards for bloods, a CT scan, an MRI scan, breast biopsies and a bone scan. He talked about me having two cycles of FEC chemotherapy (5-fluorouracil, epirubicin and cyclophosphamide), and then a repeat MRI. He would then do a mastectomy if the tumour had shrunk enough. He needs to wait for the biopsy result from the right breast before any treatment decision but I might need bilateral mastectomies. We discussed possible immediate reconstruction, which he would like to offer me in view of my young age. I immediately felt confident in his care and the reconstruction option made me feel a whole lot better and more optimistic about my future. I felt he wouldn't offer me this op if I wasn't going to stay alive to benefit from it. We also discussed a change of chemotherapy to Taxotere® if no response to FEC. I will also need radiotherapy and apart from the radiotherapy at Cookridge Hospital, I asked about having the chemotherapy and surgery through the local private hospital as

I have private medical insurance. I'm so glad this is possible as it would be really difficult for me to cope with having treatment in my own workplace. Walked over to outpatients with Gill to have the blood tests done and then went back to our office to ring my Phil. I decided to leave work early as I felt like my head would explode with all the information. Phil came home to me. We decided I should let my family know so I rang my brother Steve and asked him to tell my parents, as I couldn't face talking to them over the phone or driving over to see them. I feel very close to Phil and can't bear the thought of us not being together if I've left things too late.

3 MARCH 2006

I'm so glad it's my day off, couldn't have worked today, there's so much to think about. We hardly slept last night, so got up early and went swimming and out for breakfast. Sat outside the café to eat and it feels good to be alive with the sun on my face. Made me feel a bit angry too as without being too dramatic, I've always been appreciative of life and the beauty of nature unlike a lot of people who say they appreciate it only when they become ill.

As a way of dealing with the waiting we both got practical to occupy ourselves. I booked a hair appointment for a short cut and highlights, which I've never been brave enough to try before, and Phil sorted out the private medicine codes I would need for treatment permission and payment. Catherine rang me and she will tell Tim Perren (the medical oncologist) and the oncology matron about the diagnosis. I've worked alongside Tim for many years so it will be really strange and also embarrassing to be on the receiving end of his care and expertise.

Reflection

I found this example later from Barbara Clark, who campaigned for the NHS to provide Herceptin®: 'I think of my cancer almost as a gift – it made me take stock. Now when I crack open an orange, I smell it. When I see frost sparkling on a leaf, I stop and look. Before, I spent my whole life rushing.'[10] Well I don't see this as a gift and I want to live to be a really old woman with Phil by my side.

4 MARCH 2006

Went to Cathy, my hairdresser at the Parkway Hotel, and explained why I wanted a short cut. She was very sympathetic, as she's recently received treatment for a malignancy herself. She really did a good job with the colour as well and gave me blond and red highlights. Phil went for a swim while I was having it done. He loved it when he saw me and said I should have had it done years ago as I looked so much younger. My mother-in-law, Joyce, came over and it was good to focus on my new hairstyle rather than the breast cancer. My father-in-law died three years ago with prostate cancer and remembering Phil's lymphoma she talked about the unfairness of cancer in families. I don't feel like that as I can put my 'professional head' on and discuss quite objectively the latest cancer incidence in the UK as being one in three during a person's lifetime.[11] Phil talks about my 'workface' when I'm explaining health-related topics to others and right now I think this ability to detach myself from being a patient to informer is going to help me deal with it all. Another practical thing we did was to set up an answering machine we'd had stored in a cupboard for ages, which Phil won at a charity dinner for one of the local hospices. I think it'll be good to filter any phone calls and be selective about who we talk to right now. We couldn't get the message recorded without giggling and we both wondered how we could still laugh at a time like this.

5 MARCH 2006

I've no energy to write much today. Everything just seems bleak.

6 MARCH 2006

I had to pull myself together for work as usual today. I got loads of positive comments about my new short hair and this gave me a chance to explain to some of the outpatient staff I work alongside why I'd had it cut. I told Peter Selby (Professor of the Cancer Centre) whom I've worked with since 1990, and who has been a great support to me during my oncology career and my relationship with Phil. He was very concerned for me and also for Phil. He's treated him for his lymphoma and continues with his yearly monitoring. I asked if we could ring him with any concerns. Another worry at the moment is that Phil is seeing the GP today about some abdominal skin lesions that have become more prominent recently. I'm used to worrying about his health in case of recurrence or secondary malignancy and hope these are just innocent lesions. It was really difficult to concentrate at work today as my mind is working overtime and I keep thinking morbid thoughts about us both. It was also a very busy clinic, which ran over to the afternoon. Tim Perren arrived for his ovarian cancer outpatient clinic, and I felt relieved when he asked to speak to me, as I'd been apprehensive about bumping into him and wondering what I would say or if I'd burst into tears. He was very kind to me as he'd received the referral from Phil Turton and had spoken to Catherine. He said, 'this is not how it's supposed to be'.

STRANGE USE OF COD LIVER OIL CAPSULES!
7 MARCH 2006

Had to go for the MRI scan at Cookridge Hospital today, I see this as the real start of being a patient now. The staff were lovely to me and explained everything that would happen. I felt a bit embarrassed at revealing my breasts to the male radiographer so tried to deal with it as a learning experience as I knew very little about the procedure. Had a good laugh about taping cod-liver oil capsules to my nipples to act as markers! Not so funny putting one over the tumour though, as it was so easy to find due to its large size. Also had to be careful to only wear pure gold jewellery during the scan as any other metal would be attracted to the highly magnetic field. I asked for a classical tape to be played through the headphones to drown out the loud noise the scanning generates, but they played 'Pearl Fishers' duet which I love. It upset me and I wept through most of the scan. I had no idea how uncomfortable and claustrophobic it was having an MRI scan and resolved to be more receptive to patient's concerns about this in the future. Again, the nurse helped me by placing her hand on the top of my head as I had to lay face down in the 'tunnel'. She did this just before leaving me on my own during the scan and her touch helped me to feel comforted. I could hear them speaking through the head phones and they kept me informed about the timing and when the contrast would be injected IV robotically. My arm was connected to an IV pump which the staff could control from their monitoring position outside the scanner to deliver the contrast automatically.

To try and get back to some normality afterwards, I went to work and then to see my family. My grown-up nieces were really upset and I was glad I'd taken Phil's ski balaclava to make them laugh about any hair loss. I joked about how I could wear that and no one would notice my baldness! My sister-in-law, Chris, took a photo of me, as Phil wanted one to put in his wallet. I got really upset when Steve came home though and cried when he gave me a hug. I felt quite composed when I saw my parents but feel so guilty at causing them all this upset and worry now that they're in their eighties and not in good health. I'm also concerned about Phil and arranged for him to see Prof Peter Selby on the day I go for my biopsies as he's been getting night sweats and can feel some lumpy neck nodes. Surely God wouldn't be so cruel as to allow a recurrence of his lymphoma right now.

8 MARCH 2006

We went to see Peter as arranged but I had to leave Phil there as he was still in a meeting with another consultant. So I went over to the Breast Unit alone and was grateful to see Belinda and have a chat about what was going on with Phil as well. Luckily Phil met me in time for the ultrasound-guided biopsies of the large tumour and other suspicious areas on the left side. Not a very pleasant experience and glad Phil was holding my hand. I had to change rooms for the stereotactic core biopsies of the calcification on the right side. I found a good explanation of this procedure on the website, www.radiologyinfo.org.

I got really upset as Phil left me to go for a chest x-ray and blood tests that Peter had recommended following his consultation. The radiographers thought I was upset about myself so I explained about Phil's problems, as I didn't want them to think I was being soft. The radiographer managed to get two biopsies from the calcified areas It really hurt but at least it was a good outcome as she explained they sometimes fail altogether. She showed me the specimens and I asked to see the mammogram. She warned me that it was a large tumour but I expected that. I could clearly see nodal spread though, which I wasn't aware of, so that was a bit of a shock. I had to put a second dressing on the left side as it bled quite a bit afterwards (the bruise stayed over the tumour for weeks, acting as an obvious marker).

Got Phil's blood results from earlier today and they're all abnormal, but Peter has now gone to a meeting in London so couldn't discuss the implications with him.

9 MARCH 2006

We're both trying to carry on as normal, whatever that is! Phil dropped me off at work in my car and then took it into the garage for its MOT; it failed with faulty brake pads. So now I feel even more fed up with everything, as apart from all the worry and turmoil, I've no transport either. Gill offered to run me home and we had a good chat about the breast cancer and Phil's lymphoma history, as it all seems to be overwhelming me and I'm getting scared about staying in control and coping. Interestingly, Dr Roger Granet suggests in his book about surviving cancer that keeping a journal is an effective coping strategy. 'Making a daily diary entry gives you a way of recording how you are feeling and helps lend your emotions the shape of words. Often this simple act of emotional articulation can add clarity and focus.'[12] I'm glad I thought about doing this myself.

Some good news today was that Phil's blood results are consistent with a possible viral infection, not Hodgkin's thank God.

I told Gill how I wish I'd taken more notice of relevant breast literature in the past, as I'd feel better informed during the consultations with Tim and Phil Turton. I still get sent breast cancer related literature from drug companies from my chemotherapy administration days but tend to pass onto my breast care colleagues.

10 MARCH 2006

Joyce ran me to the Parkway Hotel for a swim, as I've no car. I took a card for my hairdresser Cathy, to say thanks for making me look good with short hair which I've never had before. I also saw Emma (my Pilates instructor) and explained the reason for stopping her classes. She was shocked as she's been helping me with my long-standing back problems and thought I was quite fit otherwise.

11 MARCH 2006

No energy to write anything today, feeling bleak again for my future.

12 MARCH 2006

Snowing loads which stopped us going to Joyce's for tea. Took the oral contrast for CT scan tomorrow morning and then fasted as directed. Don't mind not having food but hate being thirsty as it makes me feel nauseated. When I was a little girl if I called out for a drink in the night then Joaney always brought me a bucket as well, as it usually meant I was going to vomit!

13 MARCH 2006

8.30am. Went straight for the CT scan at St James's Hospital. It was a really horrible experience in contrast to having the MRI scan at Cookridge Hospital. I had to strip off in a draughty corridor with only a flimsy curtain for privacy (Cookridge has concertina doors in their changing areas which are much better.) Also the scanning room was really cold and I couldn't stop shivering during the scan. The x-ray staff did cover me with a blanket when I commented on the cold temperature, but then struggled to cannulate me, as I was so cold. The only good thing was that, unlike a lot of my patients who hate the taste, I didn't mind drinking the contrast, as I was so thirsty from fasting. I went up to the oncology clinic afterwards and warmed up in our office area before going for an isotope injection at 11.30 prior to the bone scan. That wasn't any better. Firstly, the radiographer was annoyed that the cannula had been removed after the CT scan. Then he then went on to tell me that three consultants were away and the registrar wasn't confident to report for the multidisciplinary team meeting. Did I really need to know that? Then when I went back later for the bone scan I got ignored when another member of staff came in and they started talking together. I wish I'd said something at the time but I didn't want to get more upset than I already was. Yes, we all do this from time to time when there are distractions but I like to think

I always apologise to the patient and always acknowledge their presence. I felt like they'd forgotten I was even in the room, or am I being overly sensitive and passing on my anxieties in petty anger towards others? Glad Gill was waiting for me and she ran me home again. (I've since had another bone scan and this time the same person was very chatty and attentive so perhaps I was being overly sensitive?, or maybe he was having a bad day the first time!)

14 MARCH 2006

Tim rang following the MDT. My right side is okay as the biopsies show just benign calcification. He plans to see me at the private BUPA Hospital on Wednesday. I dictated a letter to be sent to my patients explaining that I wouldn't be available for a while and giving them alternative contacts. I can't help feeling like I'm abandoning them and feel bad at not disclosing the reason, as they may think I no longer care about them.

15 MARCH 2006

Rang the oncology matron at work, as I'm sure I need to be off sick now as there's too much to think about to be able to concentrate and I need to be available for appointments and treatment to start. I asked about working between chemo cycles if possible and she said that would be fine if I felt like it.

I went to see Tim and felt embarrassed at being examined but he was lovely, and I was just thankful not to have a gynaecological problem! I also told him I felt stupid about leaving it for so long before I sought help and he reassured me he'd probably do exactly the same if he found a lump somewhere. He wants to give me EC (epirubicin and cyclophosphamide), not the 5-fluorouracil and also suggested I might have the mastectomy much later in the year, not after two cycles as mentioned before. Consequently, need to cancel planned June holiday to Majorca. Phil took this really well.

I met Eileen the breast care nurse and Jane from the IV team repeated blood tests. Had a terrible evening when we got home. Couldn't stop crying and feel scared. Gill came, which helped, as she reminded me I was reacting completely normally. Then got upset again on the phone as a friend rang out of the blue to ask us for a meal and I had to tell her about the diagnosis. The only good news today was that Phil got my car sorted out.

16 MARCH 2006

Better day. Went to my neighbour's for coffee and to the local shops just for a bit of company and normality. Called at GPs for sick note but hacked off when they were shut. No patience with everyday problems at the moment.

17 MARCH 2006

Phil's birthday. Not one of the best he's had! Woke early but feeling better, dozed off again after reading. Our friend Tracie rang, had nice long chat and then she came with carrot cake as a birthday treat for Phil. Picked up the sick note from GP surgery successfully today.

Had my hair done while I still have some.

18 MARCH 2006

Catherine sent half a dozen Quality Street toffees through the post in an envelope, which really made me laugh, as she knows I can't resist them whenever we get them in clinic. Debbie (one of the research sisters and a good friend) called with a lovely friendship angel. Told her I'll take it with me when I have the surgery. She took the sick note to pass on to the matron.

19 MARCH 2006

Okay morning, got stressed at times. Glad when Poulam came as I forced myself to cheer up. He used to work at St James's and was the consultant I worked most often with. I really miss him now he's Professor of Oncology in Nottingham. He brought a huge basket of fruit and joked about helping to prevent constipation during the chemo. Seems very odd talking about myself so intimately and so often to my friends. Joyce came for evening meal, which I enjoyed, but aware it's my last 'normal' weekend. My skin feels very itchy today, probably stress-related.

20 MARCH 2006

It feels really weird not rushing off to the busy Monday morning renal cancer clinic as usual. I rang and left a message for Gill and the girls in the office. Finished Gloria Hunniford's book. Phil didn't want me to continue reading it, but I found it quite comforting as I hadn't realised Caron Keating had refused standard treatments before she died. Went to aqua aerobics and told some of the group about me and quite a few of the ladies have breast cancer experience themselves or in their family. It's getting easier to tell people but their reaction is quite interesting, ranging from dismissive as in 'you'll be fine' or very interested in my potential treatment. I feel strange talking about myself like this.

21 MARCH 2006

First chemo today. Okay, but worried about epirubicin extravasating (leaking) until it was all in safely. I tried to relax with the IV nurse, as I didn't want to make her nervous in dealing with me. I remember giving chemo to doctors and nurses during my IV team days and it was always a relief to have a successful first cannulation. Used the cold cap to try and minimise any alopecia (hair loss). In the *Penguin Cold Cap System* information they state that it works by narrowing blood vessels beneath the skin, which reduces the amount of chemotherapy reaching the hair follicles, and also reduces potential damage to them by slowing the metabolism due to the low temperature (www.msc-worldwide.com).

I knew all this before, but I hadn't realised quite how tight and cold the caps were, so very glad when the time was up as I felt chilled all over. Still, worth it if it works. Gill called in the afternoon, felt okay but took extra Maxolon® as well as dexamethasone and granisetron, as I'm determined not to vomit. Urine very pink when I went to the loo. I'd forgotten about that side effect of the epirubicin, so drank lots to dilute it and make sure it wasn't cystitis from the cyclophosphamide.

22 MARCH 2006

I woke up at 3 am in a cold sweat. Felt horrible but not sick. Phil brought me ginger biscuits and anti-emetics before he went to work. Thankfully I managed to get back to sleep. Spent most of the day writing cards and on the phone to friends. Very difficult finding the right way to tell them. Rang the Robert Ogden Macmillan Centre at St James's to make HAT appointment (Head Art Therapy), in case the cold cap doesn't work and I need a wig and scarves.

Sent leaving form to Leeds University, as I can't continue with the postgraduate Masters' programme I was doing part-time. I certainly couldn't concentrate on the exam that's due soon. I feel so upset at having to put my life and plans on hold while all this is dealt with.

23 MARCH 2006

Bad night again, woke up with a cold sweat but dozed off again. Went to aqua aerobics, tiring but enjoyed it and had my hair done again along with Reiki from Cathy. I thought she was just doing a normal hair massage but since her illness she's got interested in complementary therapies. Not sure about effects but certainly felt more relaxed afterwards. Found lovely flowers on the doorstep when I got home, from Palliative Care Team (PCT) colleagues. Walked to the local shop to post thank you card, quite breathless coming back and felt nauseated. More calls from friends, glad they know about me, as I need all their support right now.

24 MARCH 2006

Wilma came and took me to my parents. Good to see them and explain more about the chemotherapy. They were pleased to catch up with Wilma too as they've known her since we started training in 1975. Enjoyed Thai takeaway at night but I drank less beer and wine than usual. Phil had the abdominal skin lesions removed at GP surgery.

25 MARCH 2006

Went to the supermarket with Phil. His belly's a bit sore from yesterday. Took the last dexamethasone today, surprised at my lack of energy and had to keep sitting down during shopping. Joyce picked up our ironing which I was really grateful for. Just to add insult to injury my period started (didn't realise at the time that this would be the last as the menopause kicked in with a vengeance after the chemo), and I'm constipated despite taking aperients, so this doesn't help me feel any better generally.

26 MARCH 2006

I feel awful today with dysmenorrhoea and lethargy so stayed in bed. Gill called with sea bands to try to prevent nausea during chemo. No phone calls today and quite glad not to have to talk.

27 MARCH 2006

Feel a bit better, went to aqua aerobics. Managed okay and enjoyed relaxing in the steam room. I was rotten to my parents on the phone, couldn't be bothered talking to them. Catherine came and Suzanne (another research sister I work with) rang with patient messages which are really sweet.

28 MARCH 2006

Went to HAT appointment and got wig sorted, perfect match for my current short style and colour. It felt quite odd though and I felt a bit detached as I tried it on and saw myself in the mirror. It was a bit like being an actress and changing my persona for a film. Saw PCT lot, gave me lovely necklace and earrings. This may be an awful time but everyone's kindness is brilliant. My throat and backside are a bit sore today, hope my blood count's okay.

29 MARCH 2006

Lovely flowers arrived from Mark and Keri. Had a good chat with a research colleague who has been through breast cancer treatment herself. Told her about my fear of lymphoedema as she's been left with it and I really don't want any visible reminder when it's all over. Throat a bit better, backside awful, definite haemorrhoids, time to bring out the Anusol®!

30 MARCH 2006

Went shopping, message from Belinda on answer machine about my bone scan result and need lumbar spine x-rays as there's a suspicious area showing up that could be a metastasis. Had a wobbly moment thinking all my back problems were due to tumour spread but then rationalised that I'd have known about the lump much sooner as I've had back problems for more than a decade. I've also had less pain since I saw a Podiatrist who suggested I wear a heel raise on the left side as my left leg is 1.7cm shorter than my right. So all my life I've been walking lop-sided, putting strain on my joints. I went to the x-ray department and told them about my long-term back problems and shorter left leg. There was a student radiographer who worked alongside the radiographer so I concentrated on what she was being taught about positioning, etc. I felt quite calm having the extra x-rays and decided that it wasn't a metastasis by the end of them but still relieved to get home and obviously Phil's worried until we know for sure.

NO SECRETS LEFT NOW

1 APRIL 2006

Stayed in all day. Painful backside and beginning to lose pubic hair, hope it's not the start of all my hair falling out. Told Phil about the piles and pubes so he knows why I'm so miserable! We have no secrets left now and I'm usually quite prudish about my own bodily functions. I got really weepy looking out at the garden and wondering if I'd be OK to see it next year depending on extent of disease. More friends rang and promised to tell others to save me contacting them.

2 APRIL 2006

We went out for lunch to friends. Good to be with their kids and forget about problems just for a short while.

3 APRIL 2006

Nadir today. Was going to go shopping after, but white count (WC) 1.5 with 0.1 neutrophils, so I was told to go straight home and not mix with the public, as I'm at risk of picking up any infection. Have to start growth factor G-CSF, Neulasta® subcutaneous injections and prophylactic oral antibiotics. Not worried about self-injecting as I had to self-inject both subcutaneous and intra-muscular injections during the IVF treatment. Next chemo arranged with blood test and a consultation with Tim the day before. Hopefully my white count will have improved sufficiently to allow the next course of chemo to be given on time as I don't want any delays in treatment that risk the tumour growing.

Lovely flowers delivered from our good friend Ann. Not a good evening though, fell out with Phil when he got home; suddenly feel awful, pains in legs and back, probably due to G-CSF as it can cause bone pains.[13] I've lectured others about side effects of growth factors so knew about potential joint pains but no idea how painful they could be. This is another lesson for me to learn for my future patient care. I couldn't be bothered with phone calls so let them go onto the answer machine.

4 APRIL 2006

I woke up at 1am, crying with pain in legs and hips. Took co-dydramol and eventually went back to sleep. My nieces came for lunch, brought wine and seeing them and a glass or two helped to cheer me up. Prof Selby sent message for Phil to have repeat bloods and follow up appointment next week. I had to take more co-dydramol as aches and pains back with a vengeance. Scalp feeling really sore and hair coming out when I rubbed it. Sad, but expected it really as the epirubicin dose was high and didn't really think the cold cap would work for me.

5 APRIL 2006

Better night's sleep but feel lonely today. Last G-CSF today and I'm really glad. More hair coming out, so just sat in the lounge gathering it in my hands and put it in the waste bin. My scalp feels really sore; I'd no idea that alopecia might hurt physically as well as emotionally. I'd read in one of my oncology books that 'the loss of one's hair can have negative effects on self-concept, self-identity and body image'.[14] I'd add it's also a pain in the scalp! I was a bit weepy during the evening. Phil was lovely to me and sad for me about my hair loss but insists he's not bothered by it himself and keeps telling me 'You have a pretty face'.

6 APRIL 2006

I sent my nursing registration fee back to the Nursing and Midwifery Council today. Can't help wondering when or even if

I'll get back to work, but definitely want to aim for the end of the year. Phil really noticed my hair loss when he got home and that made me cry again.

7 APRIL 2006

Went shopping for a bit of retail therapy and bought bargain hats in the sale, only £2.00 each. Really embarrassed though, as when I tried them on, loads of hair was stuck to the linings and I had to collect it off them before I could pay.

8 APRIL 2006

Phil cut my hair really short as loads still coming out. I didn't think it was very thick so amazing how many strands there are. I felt better after and wore a hat to go into work with him, then out for Thai meal. Quite funny in the restaurant as the waitress asked if I was cold and kept checking that the radiator was switched on!

9 APRIL 2006

Phil had to get the vacuum cleaner out as my hair still falling out all over the house.

10 APRIL 2006

First time out wearing scarf (bandana style), as I want to look trendy. I got a few second glances but also lots of smiles from people as if they were wishing me well. My brother Steve said I'd look as good as Kylie Minogue did in her scarves following chemo, but I doubt that very much! Called at Debbie's, she gave me really sweet card and £5.00 from one of our patients to get myself some flowers. He realised I must be ill but is being very discreet and hasn't asked what's wrong. Made me think about how this experience may change me and if I'll be able to handle my patients' cancer issues in the future or will I get too emotional?

BALD IS NOT 'ALWAYS BEAUTIFUL'

11 APRIL 2006

When I worked in the BMT (Bone Marrow Transplant) unit, we had a poster up on the wall which said 'bald is beautiful'.

It was our attempt to cheer up the patients receiving high-dose cyclophosphamide who always had complete alopecia. Now I know that our attempt to improve how someone feels about their looks is not always possible. Gill picked me up for blood tests and lunch out. I've hardly any hair left now, so it's horrible looking at myself in the mirror, but she said I looked good in my red bandana. Nadir result is better this time, WC 3.1, neutrophils 1.4, so OK for next chemo.

Saw Tim later. The lump is a bit smaller, so to continue with another cycle of EC then to have a repeat MRI scan. Possibly 2x more cycles of EC then switch to Taxotere® and Herceptin®, as the tumour is Human Epidermal growth factor Receptor 2 (HER2) positive. (I've read in the Roche booklet that this is a protein produced by 25% of women with breast cancer.)[15] I've got to have 8x chemo cycles in total and then surgery. This threw me a bit as I was expecting surgery sooner.

12 APRIL 2006

Second chemo today. I had to be cannulated twice and then tried to relax during the epirubicin. I didn't bother with the cold cap, as I'm practically bald now. I got a very tight feeling in my head during the cyclophosphamide. Eileen came to talk during the chemo. Part of me wanted distracting from concern of extravasation, but I also wanted to watch the bolus delivery discreetly. I didn't want to make the nurse nervous but I kept one eye on my hand as she was injecting the epirubicin through the IV drip tubing to make sure there was no swelling and that all the drug was going into the vein.

So glad to get home and lie down but vomited in the afternoon. I should have taken extra Maxolon®, as I didn't feel great when I got home. Can't pretend I wouldn't mind losing some weight though, so not bothered about lack of appetite. Hope I feel better tomorrow as we're supposed to be going to see *Little Britain* in Sheffield (I bought tickets as part of Phil's Christmas present).

13 APRIL 2006

Stayed in bed longer than usual and feel less nauseated. Decided to take regular Maxolon®. Started G-CSF 24 hours after chemo, will need this each cycle now as my counts went so low with first lot. Tim thinks I'll be at risk of my white cells being suppressed with each chemo now and I don't want to pick up infections on top of everything else.

We went to the Sheffield Arena with Steve and Chris and my nieces and nephews-in-law and really enjoyed *Little Britain*. It's true that 'laughter is the best medicine.' I felt quite an affinity with Matt Lucas and his alopecia and was surprised I felt okay wearing my scarf in such a huge crowd. It's funny, since losing my hair, I don't feel right in the wig I chose. It makes me feel old and seems too 'bouffant'. Just too much hair I suppose.

14 APRIL 2006

Good Friday today. Phil went into work later, so I stayed in bed till midday. No energy at all, just rested on the sofa till I managed to get into the bath early evening. More problems with constipation and got Indian takeaway in desperation! Poor night's sleep as took co-danthramer and had to get up to the loo or was it the curry? My throat's a bit sore again.

15 APRIL 2006

I feel better today and went out to the café with Phil. I enjoyed a late breakfast but sat near the door as felt a bit nauseated and worried about vomiting in public! It's like having a permanent hangover.

I asked Phil to cut remaining few strands of hair really short. I asked if he thought I looked like the beautiful singer Sinead O'Connor but he said I looked more like Matt Diskin who's one of the Rhino's rugby players who has a shaved head! My doctor friend Ann called in the afternoon with a relaxation CD, trashy novel and chocolate. Interestingly I never lost my appetite for chocolate! Went out to Tracie and Dean's later and they were very understanding about my lack of appetite and fatigue, so we left early. Couldn't sleep but tried to relax and good to lie in the dark and try to shut out my thoughts.

16 APRIL 2006

I feel better so put the anti-emetics and Anusol® away. I've got a nasty taste in my mouth though, a bit metallic. I guess it's due to the cyclophosphamide side effects as it's one of the chemotherapy drugs that causes taste changes.[16]

17 APRIL 2006

Went into work with Phil and then onto Steve's. Had a lovely meal but very tired and needed to get home as suffering with bowel problems again and didn't want to have to explain my embarrassing side effects.

18 APRIL 2006

Went for a swim. Couldn't do much as so tired, but enjoyed stretching in the water. I wore a bandana in the pool and got asked if I'd had a bad haircut or was I having chemo? I told this lady about the chemo and she then told me about her breast cancer years ago and that I'd be fine. I want to believe this but think I'll feel more confident post-surgery. I felt really tired in the evening, couldn't be bothered talking to poor Phil who's done nothing wrong, and I went to bed early to just be on my own.

19 APRIL 2006

I've not much to say as today has been dominated by pain and bleeding piles.

20 APRIL 2006

Up early to see Prof Peter Selby with Phil. Thankfully his repeat blood tests are all normal so he must have had a virus and it was just bad timing with all that was going on with me. It was nice to see everyone at work, but stayed away from the patient areas, as I'm not ready to see them yet.

Stopped at chemists to get suppositories. Stupidly embarrassed about buying them and know I should probably let Tim know as I've got regular rectal bleeding now. Another doctor friend, Dawn, rang so told her about my problems and she completely understood the embarrassment factor. She suggested I take a larger dose of co-danthramer and get some lignocaine gel.

Another friend, Ruth, rang at night and she got really angry about the breast cancer as she commented what a healthy lifestyle I led (apart from the wine perhaps!). She knows I eat healthily though and exercise most days. We talked about me not having children. (I'd tried three IVF cycles of treatment with Phil just after we got married in 1995, and although I got pregnant twice, I miscarried both times.) I have wondered if this could have contributed to the breast cancer but thought ovarian cancer was more of a risk and there doesn't seem to be clear evidence about this.[17] I have read about other women who believed their fertility treatment caused their breast cancer but I don't see the point in dwelling on it as no one knows for sure. Justine Picardie wrote an article for the *Daily Mail* about her belief that her sister's breast cancer was caused by fertility treatment, and also comments about the presenter Paul Merton's wife Sarah dying from breast cancer after finishing IVF too.[18]

'LADIES WHO LUNCH'

21 APRIL 2006

Wilma picked me up for lunch. Taste still a bit odd, but good to be out with her and talked non-stop as always! Tried the chemist for some lignocaine gel but told it's prescription only so will have to wait until after the weekend. Our friends Tony and Ann came down from Scotland. We went out for a Chinese and then on to the Leeds Rhinos rugby league match but stayed for the first half only as I felt too tired to stand for longer. I hate feeling like this.

22 APRIL 2006

Lazy day, spent most of it feeling a bit sorry for myself.

23 APRIL 2006

Went out for lunch with family and friends, certainly true that good company helps you to forget about things and it's also a beautiful sunny day.

24 APRIL 2006

Rang BUPA Hospital and spoke to Jane from the IV team about the lignocaine gel prescription. She suggested my GP but will let Tim know about my problems so at least that saves me the embarrassment of telling him. I rang the GP and she agreed to prescribe without consultation, but suggested Proctosedyl® gel. Tried to set off to the surgery then my car wouldn't start so had to get the AA out for a new battery. Thank goodness for Homestart! Finally got to the surgery and glad to get home to start using the gel.

25 APRIL 2006

Decided to go out to the café and local shops as feel a bit more energetic. Angela the matron rang from St James's and we had a long chat about my expectations of getting back to work. Realise now there's no way I could work in-between the chemo cycles.

26 APRIL 2006

Follow-up MRI scan today. Not weepy this time and knew what to expect. I had a look through Yorkshire Dales cottage brochures when I got home. Hopefully we can have a short break away soon.

27 APRIL 2006

Wilma picked me up again, joked about her becoming my chauffeur! We went to the Roundhay Park café. It's a beautiful sunny day and I feel much better.

28 APRIL 2006

Debbie called with cards and present from work. She cheered me up as I'm feeling a bit tired today and had a bad night's sleep again last night and can't work out why. Just can't seem to switch off my thoughts once I get to bed. I also do exactly the opposite of my own advice to patients which is to 'think about getting through this week and don't project too far in the future'. All I can think about is whether I'll be around to collect my flippin' pension after working all these years!

29 APRIL 2006

Good day, called at Steve's and my parents before going onto 60th birthday party for Phil's work colleague. I'm getting more used to others seeing my new look now and I'm grateful for collecting so many scarves over the years, as I quite enjoy co-ordinating them with my outfits.

30 APRIL 2006

Wilma's for lunch and she gave me a lovely strappy top. Will have to stay slim to wear it, so good incentive! I feel fine today.

1 MAY 2006

Bank Holiday but no different to me as every day seems like a holiday! Went to Mark and Keri's in York. Really good to see them but felt uneasy and a bit detached from the conversation as thinking about seeing Tim and the MRI result later this week. My back and legs are very itchy again. Must be stress-related, as I can't see any rash and my skin always reacts in this way when I worry either consciously or subconsciously. I'm just hoping I don't get any eczema again that I've suffered from periodically since being a little girl.

2 MAY 2006

Took my wig to Cathy for a restyle. She thinned it down a bit and I feel it suits me better now. Wore it to the local shops and it's good to blend in with everyone, as no-one gave me a second glance like they do when I wear a scarf. Still feels like I'm older in it though, and don't think I'll wear it much.

THE CHEMOTHERAPY ISN'T WORKING

3 MAY 2006

Important day. Phil met me for Tim's appointment for the MRI result. Tim said I'd been discussed at the Breast Multidisciplinary Team meeting. The MRI showed little change in tumour size (still 6.5cms × 4.5cms I think, my mind goes blank when I hear any statistics), so need treatment change from EC to Taxotere® and

Herceptin®. I need approval from my insurers for these expensive drugs, so can't have the next treatment as arranged. I also need to have a cardiac ultrasound prior to the Herceptin®. It's routine to have them three monthly throughout the Herceptin® treatment as it can cause cardiac problems. According to the package leaflet it can cause heart failure. I also need pre-medication with dexamethasone prior to the Taxotere® to prevent any adverse reaction. So booked in as a day case to receive both drugs and stay for observation on Monday 8th May, which is Joaney's 81st birthday.

4 MAY 2006

The ultrasound was OK but it hurt a bit lying on my left side. The radiographer told me the ultrasound result looked fine as I was a little anxious about my cardiac function anyway due to my family history of cardiac disease (including hypertension, cerebrovascular accidents and myocardial infarctions). I always thought I would suffer with some sort of cardiac deficiency as I got older, and this has always been the driving force behind me attempting to stay healthy with a good diet and regular exercise. I didn't expect to get cancer.

5 MAY 2006

Went to the supermarket on my own and really missed Wilma's help. Saw a nursing friend from Cookridge Hospital and she said loads of people sent their best wishes. All the cards, flowers, presents and calls have really helped me through the darker times. Lovely sunny day so sat out in the garden with loads of sun cream on. My parents rang and I got a bit exasperated with them as they didn't grasp the reasons for change of treatment. It's difficult talking on the phone sometimes, as Joaney's deaf as a result of streptomycin treatment for tuberculosis in the 1940s. I wish they lived a bit nearer so I could see them more often and explain things face to face.

Went to the Rhinos rugby match. My back was aching but good to shout at the referee. Cutting back on wine this weekend as I've read Taxotere® can affect liver enzymes too.[19]

6 MAY 2006

Lovely sunny day. Sat out with Phil so didn't bother with a scarf. We had a laugh about putting sun cream on my head!

7 MAY 2006

I started the pre-med with dexamethasone. Phil not feeling well today, aching and coughing, but I couldn't be bothered sympathising. It's awful to be so selfish but can't seem to summon up any empathy for anyone else at the moment.

8 MAY 2006

I couldn't sleep last night, presumably due to the steroids. Couldn't stop my brain working overtime or get comfortable and blood 'whooshing' in my ears all night. Phil picked me up for the appointment on the ward and called for another sick note from the GP on the way to BUPA Hospital. Disappointed when we got to the ward, as they've not received the insurance permission to pay for the Herceptin®. The last thing I need is a dispute over the cost of the drug. Pop had even offered to help us with money if we have to fund it ourselves. Explained that Tim was sending the insurers the latest research evidence to support the request. Consequently, I hoped it wouldn't be a problem.

Anyway just received Taxotere® today, despite Tim requesting that I have both drugs together. Also needed three attempts at cannulation before it was successful and the infusion was quite painful, or am I getting softer? Without the Herceptin® and observation we were home much earlier than planned but hopefully I will have both drugs on the 30th May. The IV team promised the funding issue should be sorted by the next chemo cycle. Although it was annoying about not having the Herceptin® as planned, I was quite relieved to have more chemo today as conscious of delay since last EC and don't want the chance of any new tumour growth. I see the Taxotere® as the main tumour killer and I'm regarding the Herceptin® as a safeguard against any disease recurrence.

9 MAY 2006

Slept better. Nice catch-up calls from friends and good to talk to them. My niece came for lunch and stayed all afternoon and it was lovely to have her company. I started back on the G-CSF injections.

10 MAY 2006

Steve called for coffee as he was working locally. We sat out in the sun but I'm very conscious of spots on my neck and back, pre-sumably as a result of the steroids I'm taking. This is not helping me to feel any better about myself now I'm bald as well. Started with awful bone pains by the evening and felt really weepy again. Awful night sweats, so couldn't sleep.

11 MAY 2006

Very achy today. Rang IV team for advice and told OK to take regular paracetamol. I was glad when a friend called and had a bit of diversion from thinking about myself. Too hot to sit out today.

12 MAY 2006

Went into work in my wig and got a good reaction. Good chat with the matron, checked my emails and post in the office and felt good to be back in familiar territory.

13 MAY 2006

Awful day. Couldn't sleep with pain last night so got up at 4am and lay on the sofa. Went back to bed till early evening and finally got up to go to Gill and Alistair's for a meal. Felt better once there and could really be myself and moan about my aches and pains. Took co-dydramol and herbal sleeping tablets once home. Still woke in the early hours and took more, eventually dozing off again. I'm getting obsessed with not sleeping.

14 MAY 2006

Went over to my parents for meal out, enjoyed the company but not much of an appetite. Mouth also feeling sore and thickened internally, like I've burnt the inside, presumably chemo-related.

15 MAY 2006

Slept better last night, but awful dream about people having their heads cut off. Then a woman from British Gas rang and woke me up at 9am, so a bit offhand with her. Went back to sleep till 10.30, bones feel better but my mouth is worse. No bleeding when I went to the loo thankfully. No energy though, watched films with my cat on my knee all day. Had a good chat with my psychologist friend Elaine and she helped me get things in perspective. I'm very lucky to have such good and useful friends.

16 MAY 2006

Awful day, nobody rang. Aching everywhere, spotty, mouth sore, nose bleeding. Sat out in the garden in the morning, but then it rained for the rest of the day. Will be glad to get out tomorrow, even though it's just for a blood test.

17 MAY 2006

Got to BUPA Hospital for 10.30 for nadir count. WC is now very high at 41, presumably due to the Neulasta®. Skin looks worse today, rash over neck and chest and nose still bleeding. By the evening my mouth had split at corners so painful to eat and wine tasted foul when I tried it.

18 MAY 2006

I didn't sleep well as up to the loo a lot. Bones a bit less achy but skin still awful and mouth sore and cracked. Decided to go for a swim despite skin problems, etc. Felt embarrassed about how I look, but luckily it was quiet and had nice chat with some of the ladies from aqua aerobics. Phil wanted to sort out holidays but got a bit fed up with him as I couldn't be bothered. I know I'm being unreasonable.

19 MAY 2006

Got up earlier as I thought my niece was coming over, but when she didn't arrive by lunchtime I rang her and she's coming next Friday. I've got mixed up with dates. Went out to the shops but my leg nearly gave way as I was walking round. Spots on my chest are much worse. Dawn rang me and after telling her about my skin she suggested I might need antibiotics. Got letter from Fiona Roberts (clinical oncologist), regarding putting me on the radiotherapy planning waiting list post-chemotherapy. I have no choice but to have both treatments due to the extent of my disease. She doesn't want me to have any unnecessary delays in starting the radiotherapy once all the chemo is over. I'll have to go for the planning process first where they will use scans and my personal cancer history to decide where and how much radiation I get. Enjoyed Indian takeaway in the evening as spicy food seems to taste better.

20 MAY 2006

Awful rainy day. Otley Show today (the first agricultural show of the season). I wanted to go but Phil wouldn't. My philosophy at the moment is like Billy Connolly: 'There's no such thing as bad weather, just the wrong clothes'. Got a bit weepy as feeling miserable all the time and talked to Phil about my worries. We went out to Harrogate and bought wedding voucher for Carolyn (a nursing friend) from us all in the office at work. White wine and chocolate tasted okay in the evening and that cheered me up.

21 MAY 2006

Went out for lunch with Joyce and back for Leeds United kick off for Phil to listen to on the radio. I'm trying to be nicer to him to make up for causing all this heartache and upheaval. My nose is still bleeding but taste is more normal.

22 MAY 2006

Lovely Radley purse and card from an old work friend, Valerie, who lives in Scotland now. Rang the office for her address and had a good chat with Gill. Skin looks awful today, very spotty, but other problems better. Phil rang me at lunchtime, nice to feel close again. Stayed in watching films with my cat on my knee again. No energy today. Poulam rang in the evening and left a message on the answer machine. Felt guilty not speaking to him, but I know he'll understand.

23 MAY 2006

Better weather and I'm in a better mood. Went for a swim and chatted with Cathy. Nose not bleeding as much.

HIGHS AND LOWS OF MEDICATION: CAN'T FEEL THE LUMP

24 MAY 2006

Phil picked me up for appointment with Tim. Bloods done first, WC now 6.2, was 41 at nadir, so no more Neulasta®. Tim reduced the Taxotere® dose due to all my side effects, as he wants me to have another five cycles. Herceptin® has now been approved so will have both drugs next cycle. He prescribed tetracycline for my skin nystatin suspension for my mouth and Canesten® cream for oral thrush which is presumably due to my compromised immune system.[20] Still to have MRI scan and a nadir on 9th June as not having Neulasta® next time. Best news of all though, he could no longer measure the lump and I haven't been able to feel it for a while.

25 MAY 2006

Awful, awful day. Left the house at 11am to get the prescription at the local chemists. Got a real shock when I discovered it would cost me £38.00 as it was a private prescription. They suggested my GP could transcribe it, and also they would order missing items for later that day. So went to the surgery and the receptionist said it would take 48 hours to transcribe. Felt like crying by now and explained about starting the medication before next chemo. She took pity on me and said to call back after 4pm. Stayed out at the café and shops to pass the time.

Picked up the prescription okay, but then when I took it into the chemists they hadn't ordered the missing drugs in so had to go to their other shop, miles away. When I got there they wanted me to pay again and go back to the other shop later for a refund. Felt so angry at the system and inefficiency and nearly burst into tears I was so tired. Eventually after a call to the other shop they gave me the nystatin suspension and I got home at 5.30pm. I was really glad to see Phil when he got home as I felt so tired and fed up with all the hassles of being a cancer patient.

<u>26 MAY 2006</u>

A much better day. My niece Suzanne and great-nephew Samuel came and we went out for lunch and shopping. She brought me a lovely scarf and baker boy cap. Samuel was so good and happy in the café, it made me forget about my problems. Debbie called with flowers and lovely earrings and hat from friends at work and cards from patients. So, all the good things about being a patient today make up for the bad things yesterday. My skin already looks better.

Tips for coping with breast cancer chemotherapy

+ Tell at least one other person the absolute truth about how you feel.
+ Remember your family and friends might need to talk to someone too.
+ Confide in a health professional if you have any worrying side effects or new symptoms. (As a nurse I'm lucky to have knowledgable friends as I found it much easier to discuss embarrassing problems with my female doctor friends.) Find someone to be honest with.
+ Keep important phone numbers – for the hospital/consultants/IV team/breast care nurse/ GP, etc. – by the phone.
+ Keep a folder for information sheets, Cancerbackup books and any relevant press cuttings or magazine articles you come across
+ Get as much practical help as possible with prescription collections, driving to appointments, etc.
+ Write down all your appointments to share with your partner/family so they know where you are. Don't be afraid to say if you want to go on your own to appointments.
+ Eat and drink whatever you enjoy if it tastes okay, whenever you feel like it. Don't worry about 'healthy' meals or eating at specific mealtimes as they can be restored later. Prior to chemotherapy my favourite foods were salad and fruit but

during it I could only enjoy chips, chocolate and curry!

✦ Take all medication on offer for any problem as soon as prescribed and take regular prophylactic anti-emetics, etc. on time.

✦ If nausea is problematic keep a sturdy plastic bag with you, as if you do feel sick while out it might help you feel more in control.

✦ Don't go into crowded areas if you feel lousy or very fatigued; it will drain your energy even more as you struggle to appear normal and in control.

✦ If you feel well, go out for company, and enjoy the fresh air whenever you can get out for a walk.

✦ Stay in bed or lie down if you are really tired but make sure you get enough to eat and drink in any 24-hour period.

✦ Keep a diary of new symptoms/side effects and whether they get better or worse with any of the medication you try

✦ Don't feel obliged to talk to everyone who rings. Get an answer machine if you haven't got one already. Your good friends will understand when you don't feel like speaking to them.

✦ Treat yourself if you lose your hair and spend the money you save on hairdressing bills on something else you enjoy such as perfume, handbags, flowers, make-up, etc. (in my case it was all of these!).

✦ If your nails are affected, cut them really short, then you won't keep catching them.

✦ If you lose your eyebrows and eyelashes get a good waterproof brow pencil and eyeliner; it will help to restore your facial features and you'll look more like your old self.

✦ Wigs/hats /scarves can all look good but try to spend sometime without wearing anything once your hair starts to re-grow.

✦ Watering eyes can be such a nuisance, it's worth trying eye-drops. Moisturise your face well to prevent irritation from all the wiping. Buy thicker tissues that don't disintegrate easily.

✦ Be prepared for menopausal symptoms, which might happen suddenly, depending on your age and the drug regimen prescribed. In my case, after just one cycle of chemo

the joint pains, night sweats and hot flushes were very troublesome and disruptive to my sleep pattern.
+ Cuddle your pets/children/partner at least once a day and find something else that's relaxing to do each day such as reading, listening to music, sitting in the garden, etc.

THIS SUMMER I'LL GROW SWEET PEAS

27 MAY 2006

I bought some sweet pea plants today. I've always loved their colour and perfume and wanted to grow them, and figured this is the time to do things I've always wanted to. Went out with Gill and Alistair. Enjoyed the food and felt good in my new scarf from Suzanne.

28 MAY 2006

A nice family day. Steve brought over Joaney and Pop and Joyce went with us to the pub for lunch. I wore my wig and everyone liked it. Felt a bit hot and scratchy though.

29 MAY 2006

Bank holiday Monday, nice to have Phil home. Started dexamethasone again, did jigsaw and forgot about time so late with next dose and missed tetracycline. Wilma rang; she's just back from Rome with her partner Frank. They've had a great time and I was pleased obviously but couldn't help feeling jealous as I don't know if we'll get a holiday at all this year.

30 MAY 2006

Treatment day again. Fell out with Phil as he was watching rugby on TV and the house was cold when I got up. He took me into BUPA Hospital for 9.30am and, after soaking my hand in hot water, Catherine got me cannulated first time. It's really good to have her support as she's heading up the IV team at BUPA now having left her job at St James's. Having the Herceptin® was okay, and my blood pressure wasn't affected. Had to wait quite a while for the Taxotere® to arrive as it's reconstituted at another hospital. The IV team monitored me and allowed me to leave at 4.30pm. Felt tired, as I hadn't slept with the dexamethasone effects again last night. Eileen came to see me while I was on the ward and we had a good chat. Phil picked me up and we called for fish and chips. I just feel hungry all the time, due to the steroids I guess. Phoned my parents when I got home, couldn't be bothered speaking to anyone else.

31 MAY 2006

Better night, slept till 5am. Suzanne from work rang and then called round later with her daughters, Sophie and Grace, and homemade cookies too. Good to see them, as I'd been feeling a bit fed up on my own. Took Movicol® as constipation problems again and my spotty skin has flared up again too. Seems to be directly linked to steroids.

FEEL UGLY AND IN NEED OF A 'MAKEOVER'

1 JUNE 2006

Went to Harrogate, thought the exercise would do me good and wanted to get Clarins gel for eye bags and cover-up make up for scars left by the spots on my neck. I was really tired walking back to the car but still good to be out. Joaney rang when I got home. Pop admitted to Pinderfields General Hospital with urological problems again (this is a long-term problem). I would normally go over to see him in hospital, but I'm too tired and can't face the journey. Hope he'll be okay.

2 JUNE 2006

Coming off steroids again, I've got awful bone pains and feel really tired. Lovely day though, got new lounger out and felt comfy with my legs elevated. Joaney rang. Pop's better and is coming home late afternoon. Got Chinese takeaway at night with chips, which I wouldn't normally have.

3 JUNE 2006

Better night's sleep but still having hot sweats, which wake me up. Another lovely day, but too hot to stay out in the garden. Feel really ugly today, losing eyelashes and eyebrows and my neck is really spotty. Phil really nice to me and made us a jug of Pimms, but it tasted strange and he had to finish it alone! Glad no one rang or called as didn't want to talk to anybody else.

4 JUNE 2006

My car alarm woke us up in the early hours. It went off four times in the night and Phil had to get up and eventually leave it unlocked. I feel lousy today, aching and tired and gave up and went back to bed. Joyce brought food but nothing tastes right except chocolate and chips and I can't help feeling miserable. Phil is doing his best to cheer me up but I feel so ugly. He keeps telling me I'm still me, but I don't feel like me just now and wonder whether I'll ever be the same as I was.

5 JUNE 2006

I slept better but my nose is bleeding again today. Rang the girls at work and had a good chat.

6 JUNE 2006

Lonely day, everything tastes lousy and metallic. Not much else to say but cheered up when I got lovely card and DVD from my good friend Ann. Always knew I had great friends and now I need them more than ever.

7 JUNE 2006

Decided to go for a swim, as my skin looks a bit better and feel really blobby, need to shift some flab. Good chat with Cathy. My nose is bleeding a bit; night sweats really bad last night.

8 JUNE 2006

Should have been on our way to Majorca today for 10 days. Phil really good about not being able to go away and doesn't blame me at all. I'd have been really sulky if I was okay to go away and he wasn't. I'm so lucky to have him.

9 JUNE 2006

Went to Ripley Castle to the Homes and Gardens exhibition. Too many clothes and pieces of jewellery for Phil's liking though and

he got a bit fed up looking around. Also we couldn't help thinking about how we should have been in Majorca.
Went over to the BUPA Hospital in the afternoon for nadir appointment. WC 1 and neutrophils 0.1 again, so prescribed prophylactic ciprofloxacin for five days. Also, will have to have Neulasta® again with next chemo. Phil went to the Rhinos match without me.

10 JUNE 2006

Steve's birthday today, rang him and he'd just got back from the pub after watching the football and having a few pints. He sounded really happy and he hates football so it must have been due to the beer! Wish I could have joined him.

11 JUNE 2006

Nice day, out in the garden. My niece Suzanne invited us over for a barbecue. Went over in my car so Phil could have a drink. First time I've driven on the motorway since the diagnosis and felt quite apprehensive at being able to concentrate well enough and didn't want to drive his.

12 JUNE 2006

Went to Leyburn for two nights. Nice place but breakfast between 8 and 8.30am so had to get up early. Did a bit of walking but not as far as we would normally go. Got asked if I was having treatment by a lady in one of the shops, as she noticed my scarf. She was really sweet and wished me well. Wrote postcards in the rain outside one of the pubs. But the beer tasted OK. Took a thermometer with me in case neutropenia is a problem again.

13 JUNE 2006

Went for a walk on the Shawl in Leyburn. Glad it was flat, as I seem to be getting breathless easily. We had a nice meal at night and it's lovely to be with Phil.

14 JUNE 2006

Drove back via Harrogate Sainsbury's to do some shopping and found letter from Cookridge Hospital at home. Should have been for MRI scan at 11.45am this morning, so rang and explained we'd just got back home and they fitted me in at 2.30pm Phil took me without complaining and then on to BUPA Hospital to see Tim in the evening. My blood count is better, WC 2.9, so will have G-CSF for five days next week. We asked about our planned September holiday to Sardinia. Tim thought it would be OK to delay surgery for a short time and I can have the Herceptin® slightly early to fit in with the flight.

15 JUNE 2006

Not a good day. Really tired so went back to bed in the afternoon. Phil was watching football on TV and I can't be bothered explaining how I feel to him, so it's better to retreat. I was glad to get out for a girlie night at Gill's to see Carolyn's wedding photos. I drank champagne and enjoyed the food. Good to catch up and they all understand how I feel without constant explanation. Stayed out till midnight and Phil understandably a bit miffed as I couldn't be bothered talking to him earlier and yet stayed out late. But he was also glad I was in a better mood.

16 JUNE 2006

Not a good day mood wise. Went over to Elaine's with my god-daughter's birthday presents. Good to see them all. Bought high dose vitamin E (Tim's recommendation to take 800–1000 iu daily) to try to stop hot sweats. Dr Sarah Brewer, in her guide to vitamins and minerals, suggests that vitamin E boosts the immune system, improves skin suppleness and healing and also has a strengthening effect on muscle fibres.[21]

17 JUNE 2006

Nice sunny day. Just lazed in the garden reading till I got ready to go to Ann's for a meal. Lovely evening with old friends, Caroline who's another doctor and her husband Ben, and I felt OK as it's the first time they've seen me with no hair. Got lots of compliments about how good I looked, but then they've always been lovely to me.

18 JUNE 2006

Father's Day. I felt guilty not seeing Pop, but didn't feel like going over today as Phil seems a bit down and I didn't want to ask him to drive. So a dull day inside and out! I just stayed in the conservatory. Started dexamethasone pre-med again and couldn't sleep, so went in the spare room in the early hours. I made up just one side of the bed, felt cooler and more relaxed at being able to move about without disturbing Phil.

19 JUNE 2006

Chemo day. All went well, but got very flushed during the infusion or perhaps it was due to steroids or menopausal symptoms. I sorted out nadir timing with the IV team and when I got home Joyce had left flowers, books and card so rang and had nice long chat with her. Rang my parents to tell them I was okay.

GOOD NEWS AS THE LYMPH NODES ARE CLEAR

20 JUNE 2006

Sleeping in the spare bed is better so I can read and not disturb Phil. Lonely day though as he was out watching the World Cup at an event at a Leeds hotel in the evening. Went to the local shops and café for company during the day, but back for 2pm to do the G-CSF injection.

I missed a call from Tim, but rang him in clinic to talk about MRI result and MDT discussion. It's really good news as the lymph nodes are clear. There's just a bit of calcification left. We talked about the number of cycles and he still wants me to have six and a full mastectomy as he thinks I could have local recurrence without that amount of treatment. I rang Phil to tell him the good news and time went quite quickly till he got home at 10.30pm.

21 JUNE 2006

I finished reading John Diamond's book, *Because Cowards Get Cancer Too*.[22] Another book that Phil wondered about me reading right now, and although I haven't found it worrying, it's very sad knowing he died soon afterwards. Feeling fed up with hot sweats, so far no improvement with vitamin E.

My car alarm went off again at 5am and woke Phil. I knew he'd got up, but thought it was time for work as I didn't hear it in the back bedroom. I rang the Nissan garage and they suggested closing the air vents to try and stop the problem. I walked to pick up Phil's dry cleaning at the local shops and went through the churchyard. I stopped for a while outside the church and nearly went in, but the service had started so carried on and Steve was just driving by and picked me up. So we went for a coffee and it was really nice to talk on our own, as we're usually with the rest of the family when we see each other. He's always been a wonderful 'big brother' and since reaching adulthood we've never argued, although I used to tease him all the time when I was younger.

I felt guilty later as I had a big row with Phil. I seem to be okay with everyone else and we both find this hard to understand. Is it true 'you only hurt the one you love'? I feel very distant from him, tired and bloated and can't be bothered trying to explain myself. Hopefully it's due to the steroids and only temporary.

22 JUNE 2006

Awful, awful day. Very upset about falling out. I stayed in bed till 12.30 just to shut the world out. Phil rang at lunchtime and feel we've started to resolve things a bit as he's trying to understand my moods. Belinda rang me and I told her about the problems between us, as I knew she'd understand but it made me feel a bit disloyal to him. Phil made a real effort, came home earlier from work and we feel closer again. But still worried it will happen again either due to steroids, or is it my personality that's changing?

Reflection

I've been thinking a lot about some of the degree work I've done at Leeds University and the many papers and books I've read during my nursing career. At the start of my biological therapy post in 1998, I read Steven Rosenberg's book *The Transformed Cell* and I've not come across a better quote than this one to describe cancer's impact on families.

'I learned long ago that cancer presses upon families like weight on an arch. If the relationship is structurally sound, the disease can bind them more tightly together. But if there is a weakness or flaw in the structure, the relentless, unceasing pressure exerts such stress that the relationship implodes. Perhaps any extreme burden does this; I know that cancer does.' [23]

I'm determined that our relationship will get stronger and not suffer too much but it's hard at times to continue with any normality. I think I expect too much understanding from Phil. I have to remember that when he went through chemo he was much younger than me, and of course his knowledge as a lay person is not the same as mine.

23 JUNE 2006

I slept in our bed to be close to Phil again but restless due to aches in hips and knees. Wilma picked me up to get G-CSF injections from the pharmacy at BUPA and then we went for some retail therapy. We had nice cakes and coffee, then her car broke down on the way home. I walked home to do the Neulasta® injection, and then drove to Wilma's car to pick up my shopping and check she was okay. The garage pick-up truck just arrived at the same time as me. Had a laugh about a nice chap that stopped on his pushbike and offered me a lift and asked if I was a 'Cookridge patient'! I felt really tired later and had lousy taste changes. Phil rang: he's now having problems with the holiday insurance company, so another dispute for him to get resolved.

24 JUNE 2006

Nice day with Phil, feel like we're back on track again. Although aching everywhere and tired I've no new symptoms.

25 JUNE 2006

Better night, grey day though, didn't go out, felt a bit whammy.

26 JUNE 2006

Slept in till 10.30. Got party invitation from friends so replied and mentioned the breast cancer so they wouldn't be shocked when they saw me with no hair. Went into work and called to see Belinda. She liked me in my wig but I was very hot. Gill was due an afternoon off so we went to a café and enjoyed dime bar cake. My taste is okay today and good to see everyone at work.

27 JUNE 2006

I've been feeling absolutely exhausted and apathetic so I'm writing this a week later and will probably miss things but I couldn't be bothered before. I know I went for a swim but can't remember anything else is this a good sign that things are more 'normal'?

The daft thing is I now feel obliged to write something everyday, partly to have the sequence of treatment documented but also 'cos I feel guilty if I don't. I never wanted this to become a chore so maybe I should just relax a bit more about it.

28 JUNE 2006

My friends Di and Rosie rang. They've just found out about me from the party invite and were very upset. I went out and called into a health shop to get some herbal sleeping tablets after I'd had nadir count, and met Debbie for a long chatty lunch.

29 JUNE 2006

Wilma rang; she's got a new car. Had a good chat with Poulam in the evening. It's so good of him to keep in touch now he's moved to Nottingham.

30 JUNE 2006

Phil took the day off and we picked up my parents for lunch and a look round their local market. So nice to see them and I felt okay. We called for a Thai meal on the way home and that tasted fine, as it was nice and spicy.

1 JULY 2006

Lazy day in the garden as it was hot and sunny all day. I feel really tired, despite taking the sleeping tablets not sleeping for longer than an hour at a time.

'RACE FOR LIFE': I MANAGED A HUNDRED YARDS!

2 JULY 2006

Busy day, up early for the Race for Life at Temple Newsam. I wanted to support the girls (my sister-in-law Chris, her friend Elaine, and my nieces Suzanne and Caroline). Last February, before my diagnosis, Chris asked me if I would do the run with them and I remember saying 'Well I ought to' as I knew then, deep down, that I wouldn't be fit to do it. Chris said later that she was a bit puzzled by my answer at the time, but of course once she knew about the breast cancer it made perfect sense. So they were all pleased when I just joined in for the last hundred yards wearing my pink bandana. As the marshals were clapping and saying 'Well done', I owned up and said I'd only just joined in and I refused a 'goodie bag' of course! It was very emotional reading all the messages on the runners' shirts and Caroline and Suzanne had written 'For my Auntie Kate', so that made me very tearful.

Afterwards I went to the Rhinos match at Huddersfield with Phil and then back to Caroline's for a barbecue. We had to go inside though, as there was a spectacular thunderstorm later. One of our old family friends, Maggie, got really upset and emotional saying goodbye to us. She wanted me to promise to get better and gave me a big hug. It's horrible upsetting people like this. I hoped I'd sleep better with having such a busy day, but didn't.

3 JULY 2006

I picked up another sick note from my GP and saw PCT lot when I took it into work. They gave me an electric fan to use at night to try and help me sleep. I sat outside with Gill and Lorna the Myeloma nurse specialist for lunch in the hospital grounds, but my neck was hurting and burning in the sun either due to eczema or sunburn. My nose is bleeding and my eyes are watering every day now, which is such a nuisance.

4 JULY 2006

I went to the dentist for my usual check-up but he was reluctant to do any polishing, etc. in case my blood count's low again, so to see him again in six months. I really hope my teeth don't suffer through the chemo with discoloration or deterioration. I went for a swim on the way home but too tired to do much.

5 JULY 2006

Poor night again so didn't get up till 11am. Tim's secretary rang to change his appointment from the evening to the afternoon. Didn't tell Phil but went on my own and felt much more relaxed without him, as I didn't have to worry about what he was thinking, etc. Saw Eileen and arranged appointment to talk about surgery options. Tim explained about ductal carcinoma in situ (DCIS), which is a non-invasive precancerous condition that in some cases can become invasive cancer. The reason for a full mastectomy is that I've probably had that for ages and it doesn't respond to chemotherapy. Told Tim about my eyes watering and he said it's due to the Taxotere® and that they call it 'tearing' in the USA. I later found out the medical term is epiphora and can be corrected by inserting a silicone tube in the tear ducts which sounds a bit drastic.[24] He also warned me about losing my nails, as they're so sore and discoloured and lifting off the nail bed. Oh the joys of chemo!

I felt a bit nervous about ringing Phil to tell him I'd already seen Tim but he was okay about it and said it was okay for next time too if I wanted. This was such a relief, as I think I'm also worried about him asking Tim any prognosis questions and I don't want to know. I'm comforted by the fact that Phil Turton wants to do the reconstruction straight away, as I'm thinking he must feel I'll be okay to make it worth all the extra effort. We went out for a meal at night instead of going to BUPA, so that was much nicer for Phil.

6 JULY 2006

Chris woke me up to tell me about programme on alopecia and wigs being cut to style. So got up to watch it and also saw a woman on *This Morning* who was having a mastectomy with skin preservation and was able to keep her nipple. Did a bit of gardening, but then too tired to go for a swim. Phil rang, won't be home before I get picked up to go to Debbie's tonight. Had a good girlie evening. Julia (doctor friend) and Kath (research sister) bought me lovely peonies.

HAPPINESS IS A COLD PILLOW

7 JULY 2006

Busy day. Went supermarket shopping, then for a swim. Nice chap in the pool asked me if I'd tried breathing exercises as he'd seen a programme about a Yogi who supposedly had cured cancer. Interesting how strangers want to help.

Went to see the Rhinos at night, very exciting match so glad I went. When we got back home there was a message from the *Sunday Times* columnist Phil has contacted about the problems he was having with our cancelled holiday to Majorca in June. She was quite encouraging about the insurance ombudsman and a similar case to ours.

The 'Chillow pillow' arrived. It is a cool gel pillow activated with water, that Dawn had suggested to help me get to sleep, and I used it with some success (available from www.soothsoftshop. co.uk).

8 JULY 2006

I did some gardening while Phil cleaned the house. Met our friends Dean and Tracie at Bellini's (our local Italian restaurant). I was worried about wearing my scarf in case any of the waiters I know made any comments, but they were fine and obviously realised it wasn't a fashion statement. I drove Phil's car home, first time since March. Got a nice card from Ken and Louise in Australia. He's now a consultant there, but worked with us for a couple of years as a visiting research fellow. We've stayed in touch with cards and the occasional phone call, and I saw him briefly last summer when he was visiting the UK.

9 JULY 2006

Lazy day. Did jigsaw while Phil watched the World Cup final and rugby.

10 JULY 2006

Sixth chemo today, fourth Taxotere® and Herceptin®, went okay. Using eye drops now to try and help stop the watering, and Jane from the IV team told me to massage my nails, which might prevent them getting worse. Wrote loads of cards when I got back, let Ken and Louise know about my problems. Good news about the holiday cancellation insurance so all Phil's hard work has paid off about researching our rights, etc.

11 JULY 2006

Okay day. Had steroids and first G-CSF before I went to the Robert Ogden Macmillan Centre at St James's for the 'Look Good Feel Better' session (www.lookgoodfeelbetter.co.uk). I called in with biscuits and cards for Debbie and girls first. There was a great goodie bag from various beauty companies and lovely to use all the products but I was embarrassed at taking my make-up off in front of the group of strangers, mainly due to lack of eyebrows and eyelashes. The other women weren't as friendly as I expected but perhaps they were embarrassed too. Gill had left message so had long chat with her later; possibly can meet up with her next week.

12 JULY 2006

Lovely day, sunny and warm, went to the annual Yorkshire Agricultural Show in Harrogate with Phil. Up earlier than usual, but didn't feel too tired walking round. Had to do G-CSF injection outside as couldn't find anywhere private other than the toilets and didn't fancy that. Sat by the Pavilion buildings and Phil sat in front of me as people were walking by. Made me think about how difficult it must be for diabetics when they go out all day.

We called at the pub for a meal on the way home and I enjoyed wine and beer, as it tasted nearly normal. However my eyes were watering all day and my nails are really sore and my fingertips are beginning to feel numb. It's a nuisance having to walk round with a tissue in my hand to continually mop up the tears.

13 JULY 2006

Lazy day, bones really achy overnight so didn't get up till 11.30. Sat out in the garden reading and chatting to Phil and my parents when they rang. My legs are very swollen, but going to the loo frequently so ought to be getting rid of excess fluid.

14 JULY 2006

Bad day with bone pain and fatigue. Just sat in the garden and conservatory. Nails worse today and think I'm starting with a cold.

FEEL TOTALLY FED-UP AND COULD GIVE UP TREATMENT NOW

15 JULY 2006

Awful night. Got up as Phil not able to sleep, as I was coughing and restless. Went into the spare room and then couldn't be bothered talking to him when I finally got up and he doesn't deserve this. We went to Di's party at night and saw old friends for the first time in ages. I had a good chat to Di's neighbour, who has breast cancer recurrence and is having more treatment currently. Enjoyed the food but tired and cold. Slept in spare room again.

16 JULY 2006

Awful day, Phil seems in a quiet mood so didn't talk much. I got really weepy in the bath and feel like I could give up now. If Tim said I could stop now and take my chances, I would. Or would I? My cold is worse and I'm just so sick of feeling lousy all the time, and being at odds with Phil. But I'm also very scared of not getting rid of all the cancer cells and know that the chemo is my best option right now. What if I stopped like Gloria Hunniford's daughter and took my chances? There is no option but to continue.

17 JULY 2006

Bad night, Phil heard me coughing. Got up at 4am, but so hot went back to lie on the cool bed. Phil rang me later and he didn't want me to drive on my own to the appointment with Eileen about possible reconstruction methods as I feel so tired. He offered to pick me up and was okay about waiting outside, as I wanted to talk to her on my own. When I'm in a bad mood, I must remember how good he's being to me. He just wants to help and protect me, but at times it can seem a bit stifling, as I'm not as anxious about the hospital aspects that other breast cancer patients worry about. I need his support in letting me behave badly and be moody, without it meaning I don't need him at all or worrying that I don't love him like before.

I had a good chat with Eileen and it was so good to talk about myself honestly without having to think about what I'm saying all the time. Called into the café for tea and had enough energy to call at the supermarket.

18 JULY 2006

Lousy night. Slept less than ever due to coughing and runny nose. Really hot day, sat out in the garden but stayed in the shade. Joyce came and brought ironing back for us which was great. Had good chat with my friend Ruth who promises to come over and see me in August. Told her how fed up I am with horrible fat body and feeling so lousy. Also noticed both breasts are really drooping now. Eileen said that's due to lack of oestrogen when I mentioned it yesterday. Probably means I'll have to have implants when I have the surgery later. I made another appointment to see Phil Turton on 14th August. Think I'll be more embarrassed this time as I'm very conscious of all my body changes and he's not seen me without hair yet.

My Phil has lost his voice, must be run down. The last thing I want is for his health to suffer again.

19 JULY 2006

Wilma and Frank picked me up and took me over to my parents. Lovely to see them, but they look so worried and noticed my sore eyes and cheeks where I'm constantly wiping my face. Joaney gave me some moisturising serum to try and protect my cheeks, as the skin is getting red and sore there too. Also gave me wrought iron table, chairs and umbrella for the garden. Had a bit of an argument with Pop about a storyline in *Emmerdale* (one of the characters is turning down chemotherapy for lymphoma) and Pop was saying they shouldn't show it as it stopped people being hopeful. I argued back that it was realistic as that's how I felt and could easily give up my treatment, then immediately regretted it as it made Joaney cry. She said she couldn't bear losing me and of course I reassured her, saying that I would carry on, but that sometimes the effects make you feel like giving up. By the time we left I think we were all feeling better again, and I was really sorry to upset them, but then it's no good lying to them either.

We called at Roundhay Park gardens on the way home and I enjoyed being out in the lovely surroundings. Frank helped to put the furniture together in the garden when I got home.

20 JULY 2006

Stayed in the garden reading all day. My neighbour heard me coughing through the hedge and said 'hello'. Their daughter-in-law died of breast cancer aged forty and I'm conscious of bringing back bad memories to them when they see me and ask about my treatment.

21 JULY 2006

Went shopping, but feel I look horrendous with cold and red nose. My nails are constantly catching on things while shopping and very painful. Bumped into Debbie and she suggested I cut them really short. Filed them down when I got home; why didn't I think of that earlier?

22 JULY 2006

Poor night, disturbed with coughing and thunderstorms outside, so stayed in bed all morning. Cleaned the conservatory, but my back nearly went into spasm, and I just stopped in time. Joyce called to pick up ironing again. Although my nose is better, I'm upset about my back hurting and still feel like a 'blobby alien' when I look in the mirror, which is as infrequently as possible these days.

23 JULY 2006

Up earlier as Mark and Keri coming for lunch. Brought lovely flowers and books and DVDs from their teenage sons, which really touched me. Ate outside at the new table but stayed under the brollies, as really intense sun and Mark and Phil have to be careful of their bald spots too!

24 JULY 2006

Went for a swim, nice to cool down in the water and talk to the ladies from the aqua aerobics class. Some of them have quite a knowledge of breast cancer and chemotherapy through their own or family experiences. One lady's daughter-in-law has just been diagnosed, she's a GP.

25 JULY 2006

Busy day, went into work and called into clinic and saw loads of people. Great to talk to them and feel part of the team again. Called at the shops and bought presents for goddaughters and friends' teenagers as there was a good sale on at the trendy shops. Went for a swim on the way home but just good to be in cool water, very hot today.

26 JULY 2006

Lazy day, stayed inside reading, as I feel really tired.

27 JULY 2006

Went to aqua aerobics, but it was cancelled at the last minute, so we did our own exercises and had a nice chat.

28 JULY 2006

Went shopping, had lunch in the café and then to spend a lot of money on the supermarket shopping. When I got to the car I'd been given a parking ticket for being over 2 hours. Took it to the manageress and she thought I was crying as my eyes were watering so much. I explained about needing to stop for a drink and taking my time, etc., and thankfully she cancelled it. Probably should be grateful that I look so awful as clearly that helped!

29 JULY 2006

Tried our bed again last night, but got up when I couldn't sleep. Lazy day in the garden, legs getting very swollen, had to elevate them. Phil did the ironing. Used nail clippers to cut finger nails shorter again; they're getting very discoloured and ridged.

30 JULY 2006

Got up at 11am. Cooler today. Joyce came for tea. Rhinos lost to Huddersfield Giants, so Phil a bit miserable. Normally I'd have been fed-up too, but I couldn't care less about sport at the moment. Started steroids as pre-med again.

31 JULY 2006

Awful night, no sleep till 8am, because of steroids I guess. My body feels tired all the time, but not my mind. Had to get up for fifth chemo appointment at 10.30, which went okay. Hb 11.1 and WC 8.0. New staff nurse has started on the IV team, Julie. The patient on the opposite bed to me talked about losing her eyelashes and eyebrows and how well they'd grown back since April. She overheard my concerns while I was being cannulated. Got Piriton® to try and help control sneezing and cold symptoms and ordered Cancerbackup book on understanding breast reconstruction.[25]

1 AUGUST 2006

Better night, woke up as it was getting light, which was such a relief. Still stayed in bed till 12.30 so seems like less time to be on my own. Watched a sad film, as I feel sad anyway, might as well sob at the film. Injection okay, but bones hurting quite a bit.

2 AUGUST 2006

My friend Jean came over with lovely pink roses and we went to the café for lunch. Couldn't taste much but good to be out. Nice long chat with Debbie on the phone later; she's going to come over on Friday for lunch. Feel so much better with my friends' company.

3 AUGUST 2006

Stayed in bed till late, and then went for make-up session at the salon where I used to get regular back massages. Felt a bit embarrassed sitting in the reception area, but everyone was really positive about the end result. I bought the foundation as it did such a good job of covering my uneven skin tones. Feel very tired today, despite looking better.

4 AUGUST 2006

Debbie came for a couple of hours. Bone pains worse today. Nails really hurting and finger ends feel numb. I had a long bath while Phil watched the rugby. Got really weepy when he came in to say goodnight and hate us sleeping apart, but can't keep disturbing his sleep either.

5 AUGUST 2006

Bad day. Finished reading Dr Jerome Groopman's book about finding strength when ill and I feel pathetic and not strong at all.[26] Will give it to Debbie to keep in the clinic library. Couldn't be bothered talking to Phil or Joyce when she came for the ironing, hate feeling like this and hope it's due to the steroids and not a personality change. Taste, nails, bones and skin all awful and very, very tired.

FEEL LIKE I'M JUST EXISTING, NOT LIVING

6 AUGUST 2006

Writing this a few days later as I couldn't be bothered before. Feel the worst I've been so far. Sunday was awful, got up late but felt sick so went back to bed. Took Maxolon® eventually and felt a bit better again so got up and sat in the shade in the garden. Pop and my brother Steve rang and spoke to Phil. Got really weepy again at night, as I feel I'm just existing and not living. Phil really kind and understanding. I feel so guilty for doing this to him, and feel like I'm wasting time being ill when I should be doing so much more with each day. Haven't got the energy though. It's hard enough just to get up and dressed at the moment.

7 AUGUST 2006

Slept in, glad to have the day go by. Started reading one of Mark and Keri's son's classics, at least I can exercise my brain cells if not my body! Stuart's a really clever lad and he sent me his Philosophy course books from uni. So I'll have to attempt to understand them for when I see him next. Phil rang from work, nice to talk to him, as I feel lonely today.

8 AUGUST 2006

Lack of sleep really getting me down now and I look awful with scabby skin. My eyes are watering all the time despite using the eye drops. Gill rang late afternoon and then called after work with a lovely orchid to cheer me up. Phil in a funny mood when he came home, fell out over me being happy with my friends and not him. Tried to explain it's because most of my female friends are medical, and I don't have to explain how I feel all the time, as they already know. Sick of this being an issue between us. Also fell out over the hedge cutting tomorrow, as I'll have to get up for 8am, and worried about sleeping in.

9 AUGUST 2006

Awful night but got up early in time for the gardeners. Phil came back from swimming to see them too before he went to work. I cleared a bag of cuttings after they'd gone and then felt exhausted so went back to bed. Phil rang while I was in bed so rang him back later and he sounds happier and friendlier. Wilma rang and had a good long chat with her. I want to stop the chemo now. I've had enough and hate the strain it's causing between Phil and me, so glad I'm seeing Tim next week.

10 AUGUST 2006

Went to Horsforth and bought a swimsuit in the sale at Oops and Downs, a specialist lingerie shop. The swimsuit has a built-up front and armholes, as I don't know what I'll look like post-surgery. There was a young woman buying a post-mastectomy bra and she looked lovely with her baldhead, as her skin was really nice. How awful to be jealous of someone else going through all this, but I couldn't help it. Also bought some Kalms® sleeping tablets. Felt really breathless walking back to the car and hope it's due to simple fatigue and not the Herceptin® affecting my heart.

11 AUGUST 2006

Slept a bit better after tablets, possibly due to placebo effect, but don't care if they work. Went shopping and had beans on toast in café, tasted okay. Sent cards to friends and getting daily cards from Mark and Keri's three-week cross-country cycling trip from John O'Groats to Land's End. Thank goodness for them and all our good friends who keep us laughing.

12 AUGUST 2006

Feeling a bit better. Went to the café with Phil and enjoyed scrambled eggs on toast. At least I'm a cheap date, if not a glamorous one!

13 AUGUST 2006

Samuel's christening today (my great nephew). Had to get up early, but enjoyed getting dressed up and wearing my hat over the scarf. Good to see all the family together, including all the great grandparents too, but retreated into another area when they started complaining about their various ailments. They're all in their eighties after all, and my patience is a bit limited for other people's problems right now. A bit fed up with the weather too, as it was cold today after all the really hot weather, which was a shame. Felt quite emotional in the church and our friend Maggie got upset again saying goodbye to us.

14 AUGUST 2006

Slept okay, but that was the only good news, as saw Phil Turton later and we've got to cancel our September holiday to Sardinia. He wants to operate on 15th September, not two weeks later as first planned, as he thinks he shouldn't leave me too long after the last chemo. I'm so glad he was so direct, as I would've hated to be given the choice myself of still going away or risking a less than optimum timing of the operation. I rang Phil at work to explain and he came home earlier to talk things through. He's disappointed about the holiday cancellation again, but not cross with me, just the situation. Phil talked about being upset that I don't want him to come to appointments with me. I might let him come to Tim's next one. I really wanted to go on my own though, as my fingers are really numb now and I've wondered about skipping the last dose. Phil Turton thinks he'll want me to complete all six though. We had a nice evening despite disappointment, and I can't help being grateful at how well Phil's taken the news about no holiday.

I'm glad to have a date to plan for the operation though, as I'm ready for this next step. Although I haven't researched too much about it yet as I want to take things one step at a time. I've only ever had very minor surgery before and the reconstruction sounds quite major in terms of recovery after and complexity for Phil Turton on the day.

15 AUGUST 2006

Went for a swim, but too tired and legs aching too much to swim, so lazed in the steam room and jacuzzi. Nice chat with Gill, and Joyce brought ironing.

16 AUGUST 2006

Phil happy to let me see Tim on my own. He asked me about this journal and we had a laugh about potential titles such as 'Ten good things about chemotherapy!', etc. I do have to have the sixth chemo, and also can't have reduced dose, but he'll give me tetracycline for skin problems. Again, glad not to be given choice, as I know deep down I need to complete this, but it would be tempting to stop right now and get some normality back. Arranged to see him again 27th September post-surgery. Rang Phil when I got home.

17 AUGUST 2006

Busy day. Went to Harrogate but had to get back for Tracie calling in the afternoon, so had to rush back to the car and got really breathless and tired. Saw another patient from BUPA in the café, and we chatted about treatments. She'd had to stop Herceptin® as it was affecting her heart. Really hope that doesn't happen to me. Really nice to see Tracie and I had a good moan about how I feel. Went out for girlie meal at Bellini's. So good to see everyone and have a laugh despite feeling so rotten.

18 AUGUST 2006

Phil off today, raining all day. Went shopping and out for Thai meal. Tired but happier.

19 AUGUST 2006

Lazy day, legs swollen. Dean and Tracie called with bath essence to help me sleep as I'd told her how it was affecting me. So kind of them. I know I'm complaining to everyone about this, but it's such a big problem for me. Taste much better today, even enjoyed a glass of wine, which will be better for Phil's liver if he doesn't drink alone!

20 AUGUST 2006

Busy day. Ruth came with our young godchildren: Elise, Nathalie and Elliott, and we went to the pub for lunch. Not the nicest family room but the kids enjoyed the food and the swings. Also had a walk in Golden Acre Park to see the ducks and listen to the brass band for a while. My legs are really swollen and finding it difficult to walk normally.

Lovely to see them all and they brought me lovely roses and freesia. Phil was brilliant and kept the kids happy to give me time to talk to Ruth. She always stays so calm and practical and I feel better after talking to her and get things back in perspective. Feel much closer to Phil again as he didn't seem to resent being excluded while he was looking after the kids and I was with Ruth. Elise told me about her school friend's mum having cancer and losing her hair too and she was very affectionate with me, holding my hand and staying close. Felt a bit weepy when they'd gone and apprehensive about the future.

21 AUGUST 2006

Up early for BUPA Hospital. All went well, saw Jeanette from the breast care team and asked about surgery options pre-radiotherapy and potential problems with implants being affected after the radiotherapy. She explained how there could be a good cosmetic effect with the reconstruction but also how the radiotherapy could cause tissue contraction. If this happens then the implant can be squashed so the breast shape wouldn't be as good. Asked how soon I could have other side evened up if necessary, as would like it doing before I get back to work. Funny how lots of people have asked whether I want to go back at all and I've never considered not returning.

Got home mid afternoon and Caroline (my niece) came over and we sat chatting till after 17.30pm. Lovely to see her but then it started to rain like a monsoon as she was leaving so worried about her driving on the motorway. Yes, I am turning into my parents! Used Tracie's sleep stuff in the bath, and also took Piriton® and Kalms® so felt tired and went to sleep but woke very early so took more.

22 AUGUST 2006

Phil brought tablets up for me early but awkward with tetracycline and not eating or no milk within two hours, means I can't have my morning fix of coffee. Got up earlier as tree cutters outside woke me in the next-door neighbour's garden. Just watched films all day with my cat. Phil rang lunchtime. Injection went okay.

23 AUGUST 2006

Much the same, lazy day, watching films, taste going off a bit again.

24 AUGUST 2006

Nice sunny day so sat out in the garden reading Plato's *Republic* that Stuart sent me. Rang work about next sick note and had good chat with Ann about the surgery as she's going away for a while but wants to think of me at the specific time. Had really bad night, couldn't sleep, had to get up to loo several times and bad hot sweats.

25 AUGUST 2006

Tree cutters woke me up again at 10am. Feel whammy today, no energy, no appetite, and peripheral neuropathy worse but legs a bit less swollen. Elaine (my psychologist friend) rang and made me feel better just talking things through as always and she reminded me I don't need to be false about my feelings.

Phil booked Hawes for two nights in September just before I go in for surgery. He's being so lovely and I behave so terribly at times. Will we miss having two weeks in Sardinia when we are having two nights in Hawes instead? No contest really is it?

26 AUGUST 2006

Woke up loads overnight, so stayed in bed till 11am. Carried on reading Plato while Phil went shopping, as I didn't feel up to it. Felt a bit sick so took Maxolon® and Phil cooked. Tired but not weepy yet.

27 AUGUST 2006

Better night but feel lousy, sick and tired while up. One good thing, I finished Plato! I shall remember one quote from it, 'Do you remember I went on to ask what patients always say when they are ill? What? That there is nothing pleasanter than health, though they had not realised its supreme pleasure till they were ill.'[27] How true is this, though I hope I didn't take good health for granted before, a cancer diagnosis has certainly altered my future ideas on what health means to me now. I'd settle for just sleeping for a full 8 hours overnight!

28 AUGUST 2006

Lousy night but bank holiday so nice to have Phil home. Went over to parents and then to my brother's for a Chinese takeaway. Ordered chips as usual, and had a laugh about excuse to eat them more often. The meal didn't taste great but good to see them and feel better emotionally at the moment, not as down, though worrying about being an inpatient.

PRE-OP ASSESSMENT SHOCK

29 AUGUST 2006

Poor night again. Went to BUPA Hospital for cardiac ultrasound, ECG and pre-op assessment. Eileen talked through routines but I'm surprised how apprehensive I feel and she surprised me with warning of possibly waking up with a urinary catheter! I feel embarrassed enough just being in my pyjamas in front of everyone! She explained how my mobility might be restricted immediately post-op but I really would hate the embarrassment of a catheter. Phil out at night with work, so seems like a long day on my own to mull things over. Felt a bit sick so took Maxolon® but not sure if it was due to apprehension. Told Phil about the catheter possibility and he understood my embarrassment but equally reminded me if it was for a good reason then there would be no choice.

30 AUGUST 2006

Car alarm went off again at 4am; poor Phil got up to sort it out. I was awake but didn't hear it, so got up early and went to the Nissan garage after picking up sick note. The receptionist at the GP surgery said I looked really nice with my coordinated scarf and dress, which made me feel good. Nowhere to park though at the garage and had to do some really tricky manoeuvring to avoid crashing into parked cars! Then when I finally found somewhere and explained the alarm problem they wouldn't look at it but said I had to book it in, so really hacked off.

Called in to work with latest sick note and nice to see everyone. Gill is going to book a girlie night for the week of surgery. Had good chat with Pop and told him about ultrasound being okay so able to carry on with Herceptin®, not sure my parents really understand about the treatment options but they're just pleased there are some.

31 AUGUST 2006

Went shopping and swimming. Had chat with Cathy and Emma about surgery. Feels like I'm talking about someone else when I explain the reconstruction, etc. Emma knows about anatomy so told her about transferring the latissimus dorsi muscle from my back to the front. Still more concerned about the catheter possibility than the breast surgery which I know is stupid.

1 SEPTEMBER 2006

Went out for lunch with Phil and then out early evening for the Rhinos match and sat in the new stand at Headingley. Quite a spectacle with an opera singer and brass band but glad we were in the seats as felt quite tired. Didn't know we'd had our photo taken from the back of the stand till it appeared in the paper and you could see my bandana amongst the crowd (Amazingly, at another match I found myself standing next to a guy with total alopecia and was comparing how he looked without eyebrows and eyelashes.) Also couldn't help wondering about the odds of us being together in amongst the thousands of people there and wondering if he was having any oncology treatment.

2 SEPTEMBER 2006

Lazy day, legs a bit swollen again. Phil had his hair cut and brought chocolate doughnuts and my favourite egg sandwiches back home. Elaine and her husband Mick and my goddaughter Anna came for a couple of hours and it was really good to see them.

3 SEPTEMBER 2006

Slept okay but dozed off again as well so got up late. Legs feel really heavy. Went to Joyce's for a meal and had a good chat.

I'M READING ABOUT POSSIBLE CLINICAL NURSE SPECIALIST EXTINCTION – HOPE THEY MEAN JOBS, NOT LIVES!

4 SEPTEMBER 2006

Slept okay but fingers really numb all day. Went for a swim, did the ironing, boring, boring. Angela, the oncology matron, rang to let me know my job was safe after the recent review of CNS posts within the Leeds Trust following the introduction of *Agenda for Change*, the new NHS pay structure (I got downgraded). Part of me feels relieved and pleased personally but also annoyed that the Trust felt it was necessary to get rid of any CNS posts in this way. I've been reading about similar problems nation-wide in the nursing press. One report is that the role of the CNS is particularly under attack due to the financial deficit of the NHS with many being asked to adopt generalist ward posts again and forgo their specialist role.[28] I'm now wondering about when I've recovered from the entire trauma of this past few months do I want to have to face all the hassle of fighting the *Agenda for Change* appeal, etc?

5 SEPTEMBER 2006

Wilma picked me up and went with Frank's mum to fantastic nursery café she's discovered. Sat outside in lovely gardens with great food. Told her about the job and we talked about Wilma's job as she is seriously thinking about early retirement. I can't believe I'm old enough to have retiring friends! But what a sad reflection of the current reorganisation that someone as conscientious and experienced as Wilma has had enough of the NHS. She bought us homemade biscuits to take to Hawes.

6 SEPTEMBER 2006

Got packed and set off for Hawes at 11am. Stopped off in Kettlewell for pub lunch. Good room in the guesthouse, they gave us a family room so I slept in the single bed to let Phil sleep better. My feet are really swollen after walking through the town centre and it's a very small place so didn't go far.

7 SEPTEMBER 2006

My feet and legs are much worse, luckily I've brought some backless loafers so can wedge my fat feet into them. Went to the creamery, rope makers and information centre so did all the 'attractions of Hawes'. Sat with some pensioners from a coach trip on the public benches and had a rest before walking back to the hotel. They looked a lot fitter than me! Also went to the cat pottery workshop at West Burton, lovely old village, and Phil bought me cat statue to put away for Christmas.

8 SEPTEMBER 2006

Had to get up early for breakfast and didn't sleep much last night. We were going to leave early but stayed talking to the owners for ages. Could feel my feet and legs swelling as I was standing for a while. Shopped in Hawes and called at Burnsall on the way home. Loads of messages on answer machine. Talked to Debbie about work situation as loads of rumours flying around about safety of jobs and quite a few colleagues unhappy and concerned.

9 SEPTEMBER 2006

Lazy day, didn't sleep well and my right arm is swollen as well as my legs today. Decided to ring BUPA for advice about oedema as operation due on the 15th. Rang and left message for Catherine from the IV team to ring me back.

10 SEPTEMBER 2006

Phil up early came in for a cuddle which was really nice, says he misses me. Nice day, went in the garden but Phil unsettled, couldn't relax, hope he's not worrying too much. Realised Catherine's on holiday so left another message. Got upset at night in the bath as I looked at my breasts and realised it's the last weekend of being whole and 'still me'. Phil seemed better in the evening and I'm really trying not to upset him.

11 SEPTEMBER 2006

First time driving for ages, went to BUPA Hospital for blood tests and MRSA swabs pre-op. Got upset talking to Eileen about the operation and costs of anaesthetist and surgery as it's now becoming very real to me and not in the future sometime. Hopefully all will be covered by insurance. Got diuretics from Tim to take for oedema. Lovely sunny afternoon when I got home so sat out in garden. Ann sent me lovely card to wish me luck. Better night but had to get up to the loo twice.

12 SEPTEMBER 2006

Legs still swollen. Lots of calls today, Phil got home just in time to see me before Gill picked me up. Had really good time at Sammy's Moroccan restaurant with the girls in the evening and had four bottles of wine between four of us! This is really good pre-op behaviour!

13 SEPTEMBER 2006

My nieces Caroline and Suzanne brought my parents and Samuel and we had a lovely lunch at Bellini's. Really good to see them and luckily they didn't get too emotional otherwise I might have gone to pieces. Got a bit weepy reading messages in cards though from family and friends. Caroline said she hadn't brought a card as she didn't know what to put in it but it's clear how she feels from seeing her today. Got upset at Phil saying goodnight to me again.

14 SEPTEMBER 2006

Wrote cards to parents and friends and spoke to them on the phone. Feel like I'm preparing for a long journey away from everyone but I know I'll be home within a week or so and don't want to get pathetic about it all. Not scared about the op but scared of the change in me both physically and psychologically as I've always thought of myself as being quite tough. Pop said the nuns at the local convent are going to light a candle for me and that made me emotional. Phil rang between interviewing candidates at work and he's going to be late home so I packed my things for tomorrow to keep occupied. Taking photo of the old me with hair and normal size body, as I don't want the nurses to think I'm usually this fat blobby mess. Rang BUPA, ward two about taking bendrofluazide tomorrow and they said not to but feel very oedematous. Got upset trying to get to sleep but slept okay, surprisingly.

SURGERY: THE NEW ME

15 SEPTEMBER 2006

Operation today. Phil made breakfast for 8am. Feel okay but still worried about catheter possibility and how I look at the moment with all this excess fluid. Watched lymphoedema DVD, *Lymphoedema Awareness: Reducing Your Risk,* before I went in. This is my other fear long-term and I sent for the DVD from the Haven organisation, www.breastcancerhaven.org.uk.

Managed to have a laugh when Phil Turton took headless photos of my chest pre-theatre and I asked him if he did weddings!

Eileen called in. Phil walked to theatre with me, which was nice but could have sobbed when he left me and saw him walking away. All the staff were lovely and made me feel at ease, decided not to ask about the catheter but wait and see when I woke up.

Quite a while in theatre (about 5 hours I think) and this worried Phil as he was expecting me back sooner. Felt really sick when being wheeled back to the room but lovely to see Phil and he'd brought vases from home to put gorgeous flowers in my room. He reassured me I looked okay, as I was worried my scarf might have slipped. Told him I was okay to leave, as I didn't want him driving home and being too tired. I had to have half hourly observations overnight so not much sleep and surprised how immobile I was, could only move my head! When I could focus properly realised I had Flotron on both legs, two cannulae and IV infusion in right hand including PCAS. Also had nasal cannulae with oxygen, four drains inserted in my back and axilla, an elasticated strap around my chest and the dreaded catheter in situ! At least I was anaesthetised when it was inserted, also as time went on I was glad I didn't need to get out to the loo as it wouldn't have been very easy.

16 SEPTEMBER 2006

Phil Turton called in early. He'd seen me in recovery last night but I don't remember that. He told me he was very pleased with the op but he had to use a small implant as well as the latissimus dorsi reconstruction, but he'd managed to do the skin sparing method (This didn't register with me till much later in the week when I realised I still had my old cleavage with no scarring, as I was expecting a wedge shaped scar over my chest.) I was very grateful to see a nice breast shape under the gown and dressing, but feel huge and uncomfortable, cannula hurting a bit and feel such a wimp.

Phil came in at lunchtime after he'd got through loads of enquiries about me from family and friends. I hoped I looked okay, as I'd freshened up a bit thanks to the nurses helping me with a bed bath. (How many times have I helped patients and not realised the importance of this intimate help?) He noticed my fingers were swollen and we managed to get my wedding ring off just in time as they continued to swell along with the whole of my left arm. This upset me as it seemed so early for lymphoedema and I hoped it was just a short-term problem, can't really see what's been done in my axilla but I know all the lymph nodes have been removed. Phil went off in the afternoon but came back later and I feel so guilty for worrying him so much. Didn't sleep too well but observations not done as frequently overnight. My room has to be kept very warm though and have to have extra covers over my left side with frequent checks of the skin temperature. One of the cannulas was removed that was sore from my right hand. I need to remember about protecting my left arm from future cannulations, blood tests and blood pressure recording as this can increase the risk of lymphoedema.[29]

17 SEPTEMBER 2006

Good to sit on shower seat and get partly hosed down but also painful to move about and need to remember to carry all the drainage bags, etc. The nurses suggested I carry the four vacuum drains that are draining blood and fluid from the surgery site in a pillowcase. It was horrible to catch site of myself in the mirror but not upset at my chest, just my face and the rest of my body. Feel embarrassed at the nurses struggling to get the elasticated surgical stockings over my swollen legs.

Couldn't fit into any of my own pyjamas so had to continue wearing a theatre gown. Really glad to get back onto the bed, exhausted and uncomfortable sitting out. Just got back and the physiotherapist came and asked me how I felt about a little walk! Could have told her truthfully but decided to stay polite and so got away with deep breathing and leg exercises. Was having IV steroids but second cannula started hurting, so stopped them. Phil called in twice and sat reading the papers, just like at home. It was so nice to be with him without any effort. Don't want anyone else seeing me like this. Asked for help to get to sleep and took temazepam as can't face another long night on my own.

18 SEPTEMBER 2006

Phil came in early and helped me get washed, hope he still 'fancies' me after all this! Gill rang and called in later with another nursing friend Rachel and brought lovely cards and presents. Felt okay about them seeing me, as I know they've witnessed much worse. My nieces and my sister-in-law came in the afternoon and I was much more conscious of them seeing me like this. Tried not to upset Caroline too much as she hates hospitals and is quite squeamish about bodily functions!

Phil Turton came and let me have one of the drains and thankfully the catheter removed as I felt it was bypassing and I was leaking urine. Not very pleasant! Drain site oozed a bit so glad I was wearing hospital gown still but guilty it went on the clean sheets too and they had to be changed again. Tempted to try doing more for myself but the nurses told me not to and ring for help. Talked about me possibly needing a lymphoedema sleeve for left arm swelling, as it's quite obvious now. Eileen, Catherine and Jeanette all called in and told me I didn't look as bad as I feel. I felt nauseated at night, but better after taking cyclizine and slept well.

19 SEPTEMBER 2006

Catherine brought in some new extra large nightshirts, which was lovely of her, so I could stop wearing the gowns and feel a little less exposed. Met Kirtida Patel, the Lymphoedema CNS, and she showed me how to massage my arm, will need to wear a compression sleeve for two hours per day and will be reviewed in two months. My brother called with fruit and Joyce and Phil's auntie came, nice to see them rather than embarrassing. Worried I'm getting institutionalised in not caring what I look like. I packed my make-up but can't be bothered with it. Phil came from work and was lovely to me, as I got upset about my arm swelling. Felt a bit rough later in the evening, desperate for a good night's sleep.

20 SEPTEMBER 2006

Didn't sleep as well, drain sites leaking. I also thought drain 3 was a bit smelly when it was emptied. Got up earlier to get washed on my own as much as possible, legs a bit slimmer but still need help with the TED stockings. My left hand is less swollen too. Phil came in after work, seemed a long day without him. Phil Turton came in the evening, can't have any of the drains out yet and he wants me to walk about a bit more. He was pleased with the fluid loss, can't restart vitamin E yet and forgot to ask why. The night sweats and hot flushes seem worse without it. Dressings all replaced and Kirsty, one of the staff nurses, was quite worried about the steri-strips on my back wound as they are making the skin sore. I can't see the extent of that wound but it feels weird, as I've got areas of hypersensitivity but also numbness. I can feel the sore bits though and it feels like a graze.

HISTOLOGY RESULT AND IT'S GREAT NEWS

21 SEPTEMBER 2006

Couldn't get comfortable overnight, wish I could turn on my side but the drains and my back wound pull too much. Threw the pillow out and eventually just slept on the mattress. Not as much leakage overnight from the drains.

It's a lovely sunny day and wish I could be outside. Physiotherapist came and we walked up the corridor, still can't get my knickers on but at least my dressing gown is quite long! She gave me more exercises to do to stretch my arm and shoulder. I rang Debbie and the girls in clinic, it was good to talk to them.

Phil came earlier from work today and Phil Turton rang with really good news as all the histology is clear in the removed breast tissue and lymph nodes. He was so pleased he wanted to let me know straight away rather than waiting till Friday when he's coming in to see me. I asked him if I still needed the radiotherapy and he said I did as further ammunition. Rang all the family to tell them, they're all so relieved. Got a delivery of more lovely flowers to my room from Ann's twin sister Mary.

Debbie came while I was having the dressing done so we had a good chat and she was impressed with my breast shape, as she could see most of the reconstructed area and said how normal it looked. For the first time I felt I wanted to get back to work as the news today has given me confidence that I'll be okay. Deep down, I felt sure that the breast tissue would be clear with the immediate response to the Taxotere®, but did think some of the removed lymph nodes might still have some malignant cells lurking there.

22 SEPTEMBER 2006

Uncomfortable during the night again and finally got to sleep early morning. Went round to the IV area to see the girls and tell them the good news about the histology and say a big thank you for their help in achieving it. Catherine off today but Jane is going to ring her and Julie had tears in her eyes, bless her.

Phil Turton coming later to make decision about how many drains I need to retain when I go home. Kirsty arranged a district nurse for dressing on Sunday. She also padded out my sports bra with 'softies' so I would look symmetrical in my clothes. We had a laugh about me looking like Madonna in her 'pointy bra' phase. Eileen and Jeanette called in to say how pleased they were at the histology result. My Phil not so good when he came, he was suffering with a bad stomach so left earlier for home. Phil Turton didn't come, so guess it'll be morning now. I fell asleep watching the TV, but then woke up lots overnight and my back feels really sore and tight.

23 SEPTEMBER 2006

Eileen called in as she was visiting a lady opposite who was very distressed at having a mastectomy later today. I could see her weeping and felt very sorry for her, as she wasn't having a recon-struction done at the same time. However I felt a bit uncharitable too as I was thinking to myself it's not like losing a limb and it's not a necessary part of the body. I felt bad for her though as I'm sure I would have been worse psychologically without my new breast straight away.

I was concerned that Phil Turton might come as I was getting washed and dressed and sure enough he caught me in my 'Bridget Jones' big pants and TED stockings with the flabby thigh fat overhanging the elastic top! My legs are more swollen today so he advised me to keep the stockings on at home. He's not happy with my back wound being too messed about with so to be covered with large Opsite dressing and left alone. So the district nurse can be cancelled as I can empty the drains myself. I have to go home with two drains left in situ after the third is removed. Interesting how the amount varies so much in them on a daily basis. The nurses padded my side so any leakage won't stain my clothes and gave me a big bag of supplies to take home. Phil rang and will shop before he picks me up and will bring goodies for the ward staff's coffee break. The drain really hurt when it was coming out, but glad to be rid of it.

It was nice to get outside in the fresh air although it was a struggle to get in the car. I put the remaining drains in a canvas shopping bag so had a laugh about me looking like 'Roy Cropper from *Coronation Street'*. Glad to get home and it was lovely to see my cats again. Phil was brilliant and helped me get comfortable on the sofa and then opened some champagne. He helped me into the bath but so heavy with fluid, my legs wouldn't bend and I nearly got stuck after breaking a plastic container he'd put in the bath for me to sit on! Got quite panicky thinking I'd have to stay in the bath all night so sheer adrenaline gave me the boost to lift myself out with great relief. Phil had to help me with the TED stockings. Managed to sleep propped up on several pillows.

HOME SWEET HOME

24 SEPTEMBER 2006

Phil brought me breakfast in bed. Now I've finished the chemo, food is beginning to taste more normal and although I feel a bit battered with the surgery, I think I feel better generally. We emptied the drains and re-vacuumed them, took note of fluid amounts and thankfully no leakage on the bed just the pads. My friend Ruth came in the afternoon and was surprised at the size of my legs. Why are all my friends so slim and petite, so I feel like a baby elephant? Loads of phone calls from family and friends during the day. Phil cooked a really nice meal and I enjoyed some red wine. Decided to just stand in the bath and use shower attachment rather than risk getting stuck again.

25 SEPTEMBER 2006

Slept better. Joyce came with lunch and took me back to BUPA for appointment with Phil Turton and he told me I looked a lot better generally. I told him it was probably due to my make-up, but I do feel better today. Jeanette emptied drains and took the dressing off my chest. Couldn't believe the result as I have no scarring across my chest but as my Phil said later it looks like I've stood too closely to a guillotine and had my nipple shaved off! I was thrilled that I still have my cleavage and felt a bit stupid that I hadn't really taken in that the skin sparing method would give me this result post-surgery. (However, I later read a paper which scared me a bit about safety considerations of skin-sparing mastectomy for larger tumours and the possibility of local recurrence.)[30] I have a lot of faith in Phil Turton's recommendations though and rationalised that he wouldn't jeopardise my overall survival for a better cosmetic result. I need to see Jeanette again before Tim's next appointment. I was glad to get home and surprised how tired I feel with the effort of going out.

26 SEPTEMBER 2006

Got to sleep easily but woke up a lot. Lots of phone calls which stopped me feeling too lonely as Phil at work. Sunny day so sat out reading Homer's *Iliad*, another one of Stuart's books to improve my mind. Fell asleep later. Emptied the drains when Phil came home. Legs are slimmer today. Wilma rang and is having an operation on her ear soon so we had a laugh about how decrepit we both are! Woke up every hour during the night and up to the loo three times.

27 SEPTEMBER 2006

Tired but had to get up for BUPA Hospital at 10am. We set off without the drainage amounts so had to go back home for them. Phil not in a great mood and I feel grumpy too with him and myself. Had blood tests done by IV team then saw Tim. Had a good laugh about my hair as he asked me about any regrowth and I told him I thought I was going to be bald forever. He wants me to start on letrozole – one of the newer aromatase inhibitors that are now being recommended for post-menopausal women who've had surgery for first breast cancers.[31] Not sure if I'm truly menopausal though or if it's just down to the chemo effects. I'll have to have regular hormonal checks. Tim didn't examine me, which I was pleased about as I'm still getting used to the difference myself.

Afterwards Phil took me to the gardens at Roundhay Park and interestingly felt I still had a nipple as it was cold and sure I could feel the area contracting. Can you have a 'phantom' nipple I wonder or is it due to a slight amount of areola tissue being left in situ? We then went to our favorite Thai restaurant and it was nice to be with Phil on our own and none of the staff noticed the drains in my 'Roy Cropper' bag.

28 SEPTEMBER 2006

'Meals on wheels' today as Wilma came with lunch and she has a gauze pack in her ear so we compared operation notes! Tracie then came with a home cooked evening meal for us, which I was so grateful for as everything seems more painful today. Phil seemed a bit down when he got home.

29 SEPTEMBER 2006

Phil went swimming then got me up for 10am, appointment again at BUPA. He wasn't very happy with me telling him to sit down in the treatment room to stay out of Jeanette's way. Axilla drain came out, back dressing left alone. Wish I could drive myself around. Glad when Phil went off to work, guess we can't be lovey dovey all the time but sometimes feel we are falling out over stupid things. I keep reading book chapters and articles about cancer and relationships to remind myself that this is normal. I found an article later that helped, about the health writer Deborah Hutton's diagnosis of stage IV lung cancer in which her husband talks about his belief that 'honesty is vital in grief'.[32] I think I'm being more honest with my feelings now as I grieve for the life I had before breast cancer and I don't pretend things are okay when they're not. Or perhaps I'm just a horrible person and I'm trying to find excuses! My brother brought my parents over in the afternoon, so nice to see them and tried to look better than I feel, as they were so concerned. My niece had sent me star-shaped cushions to stretch out my arm on. Bad atmosphere though when they left and Phil came home as he was still upset about the way I'd spoken to him earlier. Tried explaining that the hospital environment is so familiar to me that when I go as a patient I'm apprehensive as I can't forget I'm also a nurse and don't want to leave a bad impression of my behaviour. Still upset when we went to bed and I forgot to ask for more tramadol earlier so running out of analgesia, sure I won't settle.

30 SEPTEMBER 2006

Phil up really early and I was awake so he came in to say sorry, so I feel much happier that he's not still upset with me. Got lovely bouquet of flowers from his work colleagues and used up all my vases all over the house. Took regular paracetamol throughout the day.

1 OCTOBER 2006

Stayed in bed all morning, Phil came up to lie with me and read the newspapers which was so nice to feel close. Went to Joyce's in the afternoon and had a lovely meal and chat with her neighbours who called in. They thought I looked really well, so that helped me to feel better.

2 OCTOBER 2006

Had to get up early as Tracie kindly picked me up for my Herceptin® appointment. This goes on for a full year, and I seem to be getting noticeable side effects of cold symptoms and tiredness. The cannula really hurt but functioned okay so didn't complain about it. She stayed with me till lunchtime as she was meeting Dean for lunch as it's their wedding anniversary today. So it was really good of her to keep me company. We had a bit of an ogle at one of the staff serving my coffee as he was 'drop dead gorgeous'! Poor lad, with our middle-aged hormones running riot! Tracie said she'd take me anytime if he was going to be around!

My liver function blood tests are a bit raised again but the albumin levels are getting back to normal so hopefully that will help the oedema to settle. Phil came from work to meet me for the appointment with Phil Turton. He took the last drain out and it didn't hurt as much as the others had. My Phil seemed more relaxed and had a good look at my back wound, a bit messy above with the steri-strips but a nice neat scar line. The elasticated band feels really uncomfortable today, as fluid has built up over previous drain sites. Still have to continue wearing it to help maintain good breast shape. Great to be able to lie on my side though it still feels quite sore where the drains were.

3 OCTOBER 2006

Slept better on my side. Couldn't be bothered getting dressed as back really sore and tight feeling, no painkillers left. Loads of phone calls today. Can't do much without feeling fatigued. Had shallow bath and no leakage from drain sites, difficult getting out again though, I can't press up with my left arm and my legs still won't bend normally as they're swollen with fluid.

4 OCTOBER 2006

Wilma came to take me for physio appointment. Good to get dressed properly and we went out for lunch afterwards. Met another physiotherapist, Lisa, who's very nice and gave my shoulder and arm a good massage. Felt quite embarrassed as I shed loads of skin as she was massaging from not being able to wash properly. It hurt quite a bit but a good hurt that helped me to feel more relaxed afterwards. She thinks I'm getting a seroma forming under my armpit and suggested we took a photo of it but explained how we are technophobes and don't have a digital camera or phone! Got upset in the bath later, Phil pulled off more steri-strips and I feel really fed up with the pain and noticing deformity in my axilla now. Phil, as always in these situations reassured me and cheered me up. Poulam rang but I didn't pick up the phone, I know he'll understand.

5 OCTOBER 2006

Nice day, Keri came from York with books, flowers and bought me lunch at Bellini's. Spoke to Jeanette about possible seroma and she made me an appointment to see Phil Turton. Bad night, couldn't sleep.

6 OCTOBER 2006

Phil up early went swimming and came back for me at 8.30. Blew the fuses with using the kettle and switching it off at the wall. I've very little patience for anything like this going wrong but managed to fix it before we left. Then had to wait quite a while, as Phil Turton's appointment was late. He was very apologetic and doesn't want to do anything with the seroma as sticking a needle in could cause infection and would only want to drain it if it accumulated to about a litre. He was pleased with my back wound though. Asked me about walking and I promised to do a bit more and he gave me more tramadol for pain. Walked to the shop after being dropped off home and not quite as breathless. Picked up prescription for letrozole from GP. Went out for Thai meal and slept much better after taking tramadol but still can't lie on my left side comfortably.

7 OCTOBER 2006

Called at three chemists and none of them stock letrozole as they said it's too expensive. I had a good laugh in M&S as Phil got his socks and jeans wet trying on trousers in the changing room as the roof had leaked the night before and he hadn't noticed. Had to wear the new trousers he'd bought to go home in! I bought new bras from their mastectomy range and spent the voucher Gill had brought for me. It's quite difficult to get ones without underwiring from the normal range and the extra support at the side is more comfortable. The shop assistant at the till asked me for feedback and I said I'd write to the manageress. One immediate suggestion was to have wider straps as I find them more comfortable at the moment.

8 OCTOBER 2006

Lie in today, tired and getting prickly pain in chest presumably due to the nerves being cut during the surgery. Joyce came and feel really fed up but cheered up a bit when we went out for a meal.

9 OCTOBER 2006

Up late. Belinda rang and had long chat, will make me an appointment to see Fiona Roberts (clinical oncologist) at St James's in the breast clinic. Joyce picked me up for physio appointment and managed to get some letrozole at local chemist and bought a bath pillow which might help me to be more comfortable. Felt better after physio, sore during treatment and massage but nice to stretch out. Phil seems distant today, told him about radiotherapy appointment and he will try to go with me. Legs swollen again but managed to lie down in the bath, which was bliss.

10 OCTOBER 2006

Didn't get up till 11.45. Phil rang, can go with me to see Fiona and sounded in a happier mood. I sorted my clothes out and got rid of everything that was on the small side and all my tops with tight sleeves. Filled four bags for 'Help the Aged' and thought how 'aged' I feel at the moment! Nice meal at Dean and Tracie's in the evening, so we both cheered up. It's good for Phil to have supportive friends too.

11 OCTOBER 2006

Didn't sleep too well, hot sweats all night. Lousy weather all day, raining. Spoke to Joaney and rang Gill about going out for a meal, she said she'd come round later as I sounded so fed up. Poulam rang as Phil arrived home so had quick chat and apologised for not wanting to talk the other night. Gill fed up about *Agenda for Change* appeal being rejected so we opened a bottle of wine and had a good moan to each other. Also had a laugh as she loves shoes and I'd bought her the book, *Why Men Don't Have a Clue and Women Always Need More Shoes*, as a present for being so lovely to me.[33]

THE NEXT STEP: RADIOTHERAPY DISCUSSION

12 OCTOBER 2006

Slept okay but very hot again. Got up at 10.30 and enjoyed being out in the garden as it's been a lovely sunny day. Cut loads of lavender and walked to the shop but my back and hips really aching today. Phil picked me up for the clinic with Fiona Roberts in the afternoon. Went in my car to give it a run but also to be able to park in the grounds as I'm still paying for my parking permit at the hospital while off sick. I felt a bit weird going to 'work' as a patient but Sue (the outpatient senior nurse) met us and took us into a consultation room to wait rather than the main waiting area. Fiona was really nice and explained I might have to delay radiotherapy until the general swelling and seroma had reduced but will decide at the planning appointment on 18th October. Hope there isn't a delay as I want to feel well for Christmas and my birthday (28th December).

Will need 15 sessions and also need supraclavicular fossa irradiating as nodes obvious on MRI. Felt a bit shocked by that, as I'd assumed only my axilla nodes were affected but didn't say anything to Fiona, as I didn't want to worry Phil. Phil asked if a delay was necessary – would that be a problem? Fiona said a couple of weeks would be fine but wouldn't want more than that as it was important to keep up the pace of treatment to eradicate any malignant cells still around. Saw Belinda in clinic and said hello to other staff but some new faces I didn't recognise. Guess I have been away quite a while now.

Went up to the office to check emails and post, no one else there which was a shame as I like to catch up with the girls when I get the chance.

Went for an Indian meal on the way home but my car started to make a funny noise on the way and when we stopped at the restaurant oil was pouring out from the engine. Called the AA and ordered food while we were waiting. Had to be towed to a garage in Horsforth but the AA guy was really good and took us home along with our takeaway curry. Sounds like a bad prognosis for the car, as it's probably the oil pump!

13 OCTOBER 2006

Up early for Wilma to take me for appointments with Phil Turton and physio. He was pleased with my progress, told him about Fiona and he will write to her with facts about the implant he used. She wants me to start using aqueous cream over my breast area and he said that was okay. Took post-op photos and Eileen came to have a look at my new chest. Told them I was starting to see the positives now (like still having my own cleavage, etc.), rather than the negatives such as my deformed armpit and the 'fatty' pad on my side and Phil Turton was pleased. I still dislike the deformity in my axilla though and the fatty swelling on my side. Need to see him again early January 2007 after the radiotherapy. He wants me to persevere with the chest band to compress the implant down into a natural breast shape, unless my skin gets sore during radiotherapy. Lisa helped a lot with my shoulder and massage.

Good news when Phil got home, car needs a new part but it's not the oil pump so won't be quite as expensive. Decided to ask about moving back to our room as sick of being on my own at night and feel lonely. Slept okay but worried about disturbing Phil as I kept throwing the quilt off and on with the night sweats.

14 OCTOBER 2006

Stayed in bed while Phil cleaned up downstairs. Seems a bit offhand with me again and I told him to get over it before we go out tonight to Gill's. Told him I felt upset but also haven't got the energy to keep falling out. Cleared the air a bit and went to the supermarket. Bumped into Poulam and his wife Marie and had a good chat at the deli counter. Gill picked us up and had lovely meal and lots to drink. Wanted Phil to enjoy himself and just relax and forget about all our troubles. So we had a good singsong with their karaoke game and played 'Who wants to be a millionaire'. Taxi home and slept okay, not as hot.

'A THOUSAND TIMES BETTER THAN EXPECTED'

15 OCTOBER 2006

Lie in while Phil did the ironing. He seems very quiet and I told him I shouldn't have to watch everything I say or don't say as I feel I'm upsetting him all the time. We made friends and I asked him what he thought of my new breast. He said it was a thousand times better than he'd anticipated (I thought that was so lovely and put it in my 'Thank you' card to Phil Turton later). I considered going back into the spare room again as I thought I might be keeping Phil awake but he told me not to. I really want us to get closer again.

16 OCTOBER 2006

Hips and back really sore overnight, kept me awake. I guess it's the letrozole causing the joint pains. Phil rang and will try to get home before I get picked up for girlie night out. Can't deny I'm looking forward to having a good laugh instead of the intense soul searching Phil seems to want at the moment. He's such a sensitive soul and I know I should be more understanding. Just managed to see him briefly before I got the lift with Gill and Ali. Really nice to see the girls and ignored any feelings of guilt at enjoying myself.

17 OCTOBER 2006

Up early for my niece to pick me up for lymphoedema appointment with Kirtida. Awful day, foggy and raining. Took spare dressings, etc. back to ward two and chemotherapy article from *Nursing Standard* for IV team. Got new chest band as the Velcro had stopped working on the old ones. Kirtida was very nice and gave me a sleeve to wear when using my arm more, shopping, gardening, etc. for mild lymphoedema. Warned me it could get worse during the radiotherapy so it's worth trying to manage it throughout with massage and skin care but not to wear the sleeve during treatment.

Arrived home for my doctor friend Caroline's visit and she turned up with flowers, books, and DVDs. Had really good catch up and we discussed all our combined ailments as she's been off work for a long time too.

18 OCTOBER 2006

Poor night, tried ibuprofen for joint pains. Had to get to BUPA for 8am physio. Lisa worked on my arm and it felt really sore but much more relaxed afterwards. Phil took me back home and went to work. Joyce picked me up for Cookridge appointment for radiotherapy planning. I saw Fiona's registrar who thinks I can go ahead with November treatment. Gave me leaflet about skin care with simple soap, aqueous cream, not to soak in bath, etc. Warned me about sunburn effect. Planning CT scan was okay but glad to finish as my arm was hurting and marking on my sensitive skin not very nice. Also one of the staff didn't seem too confident about the measurements he was making but thankfully they were double checked by another more experienced person. Some of the measurements have to be permanently tattooed as the radiotherapy has to be very precise each visit. The tattoos hurt but very small dots and again the chap doing them wasn't very amused when I asked if he did hearts or flowers! Guess he was concentrating. Only took one hour to complete everything so went to the canteen for lunch as Joyce picking me up later. Had a chat with a couple of the research sisters I know as I bumped into them in the corridor.

Rang Phil when I got home, car still not fixed. Felt really tired so had a lie down, Pop rang while I was trying to sleep so ignored the message but rang him back later.

19 OCTOBER 2006

Lazy day. Why am I so tired? Keri woke me up at 11am with invite for lunch at the weekend. A nursing friend who I haven't seen for ages came round with flowers and goodies which was really kind of her. Walked to the shop when she'd gone to get some exercise but my legs are aching and it's not very far.

20 OCTOBER 2006

Lie in till 10.30 but legs really hurting and awake loads during the night. Joyce came to take Phil to the garage to pick up my car, he wasn't too pleased about the disruption to his day but then apologised later when he brought it home. We had a nice evening and I felt closer to him than I have for a while. I need to remember how all this is worrying him and what he's been through himself. Perhaps what I'm going through is bringing back bad memories.

21 OCTOBER 2006

Nice day, so went out to the local shops. Wore compression sleeve as my arm aching quite a bit, feels better as I drive as it doesn't wobble so much when I change gear. Sorted out friend's Christmas gifts, as I don't feel tired today.

22 OCTOBER 2006

The hairs have started growing back on my legs now but not much on my head yet! Typical, wouldn't have minded the lack of leg hair being permanent.

Went to Phil's uncle for a birthday tea for Joyce. Enjoyed the company and Uncle John's homemade wine but Joyce complaining of a cold so cancelled planned trip to my parents tomorrow. Phil a bit upset as he'd taken the day off work especially for us all to get together. He said 'you and me against the world', which I liked as it seems like that sometimes and yet at others, just lately, we can be so far apart in our reactions and thinking.

23 OCTOBER 2006

Up early for physio and Herceptin® before trip to my parents. Lisa pleased with healing on my back and thinks there's less fluid accumulation too. Nice to have Phil with me for company during the infusion. Counted up treatments and Catherine altered records, as they were wrong, as I didn't get the first prescribed dose on time. So glad Phil's so organised and has taken over the BUPA insurance official stuff for me. Called at my brother's on the way to my parents, the house is a mess as they've got workmen knocking down their old conservatory. Made me glad we're not planning any home improvements, as I couldn't stand the disruption right now.

Went out for fish and chips with Joaney and Pop, they're worried about my brother too as he needs investigations (CXR & ECG) for chest pain. Felt bad, as Steve didn't say anything to me about it and before my illness he would have turned to me for advice and support.

24 OCTOBER 2006

Lie in as usual, how on earth will I ever get up for work again? Wilma rang to meet up on Friday; she's officially retiring on 17th November. Can't believe we've worked for 31 years as I still remember the day we met during the entrance interviews. My 'old friend' really does seem old now!

Went to the local shops and driving felt okay with wearing the sleeve.

Debbie rang to arrange a meal on Friday, totally forgot we'd talked about that before and also that Phil was having the day off. Hate letting people down and also hate my memory at the moment, as I can't seem to retain things. Phil upset that I'd forgotten about him taking time off work and had a row about me then cancelling Debbie and Wilma. Told him good friends always understand but went up to bed to get away from the arguing. Phil came up to talk things through as he always wants to clear the air but I've no patience with him and his sensitivity right now. At times I feel really concerned for our future and so I was really thankful that we were okay with each other by the next morning.

Reflection

I've read loads of articles about cancer over the years and one that I found later, when all my treatment was nearly complete, describes how cancer throws emotions into turmoil and relationships can break up.[34] This article highlights several studies that report on breast cancer sufferers having impaired quality of life for several years after diagnosis. Ultimately relationships can suffer as women deal with emotional and physical changes to their lives. I've experienced this with my own patients and on top of the turmoil of cancer to lose the closest person to you must be terrible.

25 OCTOBER 2006

Sent cards to Debbie and Wilma to say sorry for double booking and being 'doolally'! Okay with Phil now. Stayed in all day and not much else to say. Went to bed early.

26 OCTOBER 2006

Phil off early to Amsterdam for work and pleased we were friends, as I hate him travelling alone and get separation anxiety till I see him again. I'm always so scared of something happening to either of us when we're apart. Guess this stems from Phil being ill again with the lymphoma just as we'd got together. He got home at 9.45pm, so a long day on my own to think about us and how I'm feeling. So glad he was safe and sorry for wasting our time arguing.

27 OCTOBER 2006

Nice day went out shopping, called at Joyce's then Bellini's in the evening. Really appreciated being with Phil and I want us to start enjoying life again.

28 OCTOBER 2006

Went for lunch at Mark and Keri's in York. Love being at their house with the kids coming and going. It's a proper family home which I would have loved if we could have had children. Had a good laugh with them and carved out pumpkins for Halloween for their daughter Laura to take to the hotel where she works part-time.

29 OCTOBER 2006

Extra hour in bed as the clocks went back last night. Went to the homes and gardens fair in Harrogate and it was a lovely sunny day. Enjoyed walking but breathless and achy. Rang my sister-in-law, Chris, when we got back, Steve to have ECG next week as I start the radiotherapy. What a family, we must have rotten genes!

30 OCTOBER 2006

Phil off today so nice lie in together. Went into the garden to do a bit of tidying up but achy and feel a bit fed up. That got worse when I rang the GP for a repeat prescription of the letrozole. Won't accept phone requests so have to write in for it. Cheered up by watching *Green Wing* on DVD and having a laugh at the ridiculous characters.

31 OCTOBER 2006

Up early for physio, last appointment with Lisa but can ring during radiotherapy if I need help. Called with letter to GP for the letrozole and asked when it will be available – possibly Wednesday after 4pm. My friend Ann came from the airport as she'd just got back from Ireland and we had a lovely lunch at Bellini's. She brought lovely flowers and amazing Irish chocolates so forgot about prescription hassles. Had last long soak in bath before radiotherapy starts.

'BURN BABY BURN'

1 NOVEMBER 2006

First radiotherapy session. Okay on my own but not nice lying on the metal table with just a piece of paper on it. Felt really alone when I was left in the room even though I knew the staff could see me on screen. Rachel Clark describes feeling like a part of the machinery and like a car on an assembly line during her radiotherapy treatment for a facial cancer.[35] I felt the same, like I was waiting for parts to be fitted to make me whole again.

I bumped into a lovely couple we know through Phil's work on the way out. They were shocked to see me there and to find out about the breast cancer but Sally is being treated for a brain tumour and so it made me feel I was far luckier with my diagnosis. She's had surgery and radiotherapy and is now on temozolamide. Left a message for Phil to let him know about Sally when I got home as I had to go out again to pick up the prescription. Chemist only had half the amount in stock so another hassle in getting the rest later, glad to get home. Couldn't stop thinking about Sally, Phil very shocked to hear the news. Booked the Traddock at Austwick for my 50th birthday treat. Had to sit in the bath as I couldn't have a nice soak and annoyed at life in general today.

2 NOVEMBER 2006

Quicker visit for radiotherapy today, they're very efficient in the outpatient area. Took sick note into work and called in to see Prof Peter Selby. Tim came into the office while I was there and it seemed odd talking to him without it being a consultation with him. Peter asked me about the journal and whether I'd persevered with it. Told him I was still keeping a daily record and how much it was helping me to find some useful purpose for undergoing the 'cancer journey'. Had lunch with Debbie and called into the office to see the girls. Krystina thought I looked good, haven't seen her for ages, so that made me feel better. Had best night's sleep so far, fewer hot flushes.

3 NOVEMBER 2006

What was I saying about efficiency? Treatment took ages to set up and had a male trainee manager in as well staring at my topless body! Felt cold and uncomfortable but can't blame the staff who have to be so careful in positioning you accurately to prevent future complications. Also didn't want to seem prudish in refusing to let the trainee see the set-up but perhaps I should be more honest about my feelings and should have said I'd prefer not. Seems like the only person I can be my true self with is Phil and he doesn't deserve all my anger and frustrations. Feel like a piece of meat when I'm laid on that awful metal slab/table. Rang Phil for a chat when I got home to get over the lonely feeling. Ruth rang which was good too as we had a laugh about me 'flashing' at the young trainee and possibly scaring him away from the NHS or women for life! Glad there's no treatment over the weekend. Nice evening with Phil.

4 NOVEMBER 2006

Lie in. Tony and Ann came down from Scotland in the afternoon. Went to Bellini's for a meal and then to the local junior school bonfire as they always have spectacular fireworks. Felt tired but okay and it was really good to see our friends

5 NOVEMBER 2006

Went to Steve's after quick visit to parents. Great time with fireworks and eating good old traditional 'pie and peas'. When my niece Caroline arrived all wrapped up in a woolly scarf and hat she looked just like she'd stepped out of the 'Wham' video 'Last Christmas I gave you my heart, but the very next day, you gave it away'. I started singing and the others joined in so it was a bit surreal singing Christmas songs on bonfire night! The good laugh we had and lots of wine helped me forget about things for a while.

6 NOVEMBER 2006

Up later for 12.20 appointment. Had an hour delay then trouble setting up again. On a different machine this time and wondered if that was a problem but radiographer thinks it may be as the seroma is settling and that might be changing tattoo positioning and their measurements on the original plan. Might need re-planning if it continues to be so difficult each day. Went to Dean and Tracie's for another meal, they've been so good to us.

7 NOVEMBER 2006

Same machine as yesterday. Better with setting up but scar area on my back is feeling sore with positioning and pulling. Had a good laugh as they were playing 'burn baby burn' through to the room during the treatment. Mentioned it to one of the radiographers and she admitted they didn't really hear the soundtracks as they were concentrating on the positioning, etc. She always speaks to me as she's leaving the treatment room such as 'off we go then', or 'last time' and this helps such a lot to make you feel supported. I guess she probably gets fed up with the repetition but it certainly helps me. Went to chemist afterwards to pick up owed letrozole, hope this isn't going to happen with each prescription.

8 NOVEMBER 2006

Treatment okay today so went to the shops and café as I didn't want to be on my own. Dress agency lady noticed my scarf and asked me about treatment, she was shocked about my problems, as she hasn't seen me for a while. Posted a card for Sally just to say how sorry we were about her awful time and inviting her and Mike to call round when she next visits Cookridge Hospital.

9 NOVEMBER 2006

Treatment delayed, machine broke down. Quite a few disgruntled people in the waiting area but honestly not bothered myself. Although I know I'm very lucky to live so close and time delays don't bother me as I've got the luxury of no other commitments. Makes me realise how difficult life with young families must be for patients. Not only physically busy but also coping with the emotional side of things. In his book on surviving cancer Dr Roger Granet describes how a woman with breast cancer hadn't told her children but they sensed the tension in the air and how they tried to cheer her up which made her cry.[36] Also I'm approaching this as being the last 'bad' bit of the whole process for me, so a bit of extra time needed doesn't really bother me as I feel I can see 'the light at the end of the tunnel'. I feel the radiotherapy is the last cancer treatment as the tumours should all have gone now.

Called into the stables by the local church to have a look at plans for a new housing development nearby. The church was open too so had a wander round and the church warden showed me a window dating back to Oliver Cromwell's time and explained more of the history of the lovely old building. Felt very peaceful and can understand how people turn to prayer and religion at times of stress. I could have just sat there all afternoon but had to get back to see Joyce and Phil as he was taking her to a cardiology appointment. She needs a 24-hour ECG and CXR. What is it with my family and their hearts?!

10 NOVEMBER 2006

Phil off today. Nice to have him take me to Cookridge and be waiting when I came out. Trouble with setting up again but didn't take as long and not as uncomfortable or perhaps I'm just getting used to it. I'm surprised at how affected I feel by the radiotherapy as lots of staff I've come across use the term 'Don't worry, it's much easier than having courses of chemo'. I can appreciate that it's not immediately as toxic to the system, but it's still a pretty intense experience. I still don't feel it's the 'doddle' though that some people have said and will be glad to finish the course. I think we sometimes, as health professionals make the wrong assumptions of how debilitating some of the treatments are. I'd like to think I won't come out with clichés or downplay the treatments with my future patients.

11 NOVEMBER 2006

Woke up with sore throat, strepsils helped. Wrapped some Christmas presents and enjoyed day away from Cookridge. Had early night as Phil tired and that suited me, as I seem to be permanently tired these days.

12 NOVEMBER 2006

Lie in, throat better. Wrapped more presents. Putting loads of aqueous cream on chest and axilla and noticed areola area looks less puckered than immediately post-op. So hopefully that will settle to give a good cosmetic result in time.

13 NOVEMBER 2006

Up early for Herceptin® at 9.30 at BUPA and then to Cookridge for appointment. Just got there in time for my appointment after having the Herceptin® infusion, then had one hour delay. Hurt me during positioning again and got stabbing pain in my left side, feel such a wimp. Rang my sister-in-law Chris and Wilma as I got their birthday presents mixed up in my current batty state.

14 NOVEMBER 2006

Later appointment today so nice to have a lie in. Bit of a delay but otherwise okay. Went to Otley for some retail therapy and ordered a wrap-over dress and had nice lunch in the café. New owners overcharged me but only realised after I'd left. Really wanted to forget about it as it was only a few pounds. I keep thinking I shouldn't fret over small issues anymore but the Yorkshire spirit of 'value for money' won't let me forget it. Phil had rung while I was out to check I was okay.

15 NOVEMBER 2006

Radiographer hurt my arm by pulling on it but he wasn't to know how hypersensitive it is after surgery. Made me think it would be a good idea to fill out one of the body charts and each patient could shade in areas of altered sensitivity such as the one recommended for recording results of radiation at www.remm.nlm.gov/Body-Chart.pdf.

Went to Otley afterwards to pick up the dress but it hadn't arrived. Got money back from café though so not totally wasted journey and made me feel better. Forgot my Visa pin number and forgot to take letrozole in the morning, wonder if the 'rays' are affecting my brain too!

16 NOVEMBER 2006

Okay appointment, still sore though but not going to whinge. Went to the café and had curry as Phil out with work colleagues tonight.

17 NOVEMBER 2006

Couldn't be bothered writing this on time as feeling so jaded, so can't remember much apart from okay radiotherapy.

18 NOVEMBER 2006

Went to Otley with Phil, picked up dress and called at Joyce's. She was upset as one of her friends had died at home and hadn't been found for a few days. She'd rung her several times and left messages and eventually rang her son who went over and found her. How awful to die alone like that. We stayed with her for a while, talking about life and problems. I felt better as we left as Joyce said she thought I looked a lot less bloated in my face since the last time we met up.

19 NOVEMBER 2006

Wrapped some more presents. Not feeling too enthusiastic about Christmas this year. Not much else to say.

20 NOVEMBER 2006

Up early for cardiac ultrasound scan at BUPA. Struggled to get good picture and measurements as my anatomy has changed since surgery. Need to see the cardiologist next week for possible injection and different type of scan. Had lunch at Cookridge and very interesting to be there, in the canteen, as a patient, felt like I was undercover as I was sitting very close to a table of managers and consultants who were totally oblivious to my presence and talking about all sorts.

Had treatment earlier than planned and saw Fiona Roberts in review clinic. She advised me to stop wearing my bra due to the redness of my skin. She had a look at a mole on my back that Phil thinks is changing. I can't see it but have noticed it's more sensitive and prominent when he helps me to wash in the bath. She thinks it's okay but should get it checked by my GP. I asked about swimming again and not to go back before January as the chlorine could irritate the skin further. Forgot to ask about the sleeve and when I could start wearing it again. Told her how I hadn't enjoyed the experience but not the staff's fault.

21 NOVEMBER 2006

Last radiotherapy appointment and really pleased it's over, trouble with setting up again and sore back. Went to the shops for retail therapy and bought skincare products, as I feel old and ugly. I may not have spent much on my hair this past few months but have certainly made up for it on make-up, etc!

22 NOVEMBER 2006

Had lie in but slept better. Nice to have free time again with no appointments to get to on time. Joints really sore and felt cold all day despite having the heating on at home.

23 NOVEMBER 2006

Wilma picked me up and we went to Harrogate. Amazingly didn't spend anything apart from coffee and lunch. Enjoyed looking round though and Wilma's company of course.

24 NOVEMBER 2006

Phil off today, he needs the break, wish he would take longer but he feels it's a waste to just be at home. Lousy weather, went to the café and the supermarket. Saw one of the ladies I talk to when swimming. She gave me a hug and said she'd missed me. Skin quite red and sore today at irradiated sites, using loads of aqueous cream, looks and feels like sunburn, especially over supraclavicular fossa area.

25 NOVEMBER 2006

Walked to the café, nice day but cold. My side and breast feel really sore and tight. Sat outside under the canopy and pretended we were in Paris. Phil saying some lovely things today about me being his whole world and how good we are together. Hope this means we can stop having disagreements about how I'm dealing with it all and get back the closeness we've always had.

26 NOVEMBER 2006

Wrapped some more Christmas presents, so much for cutting down this year, seems like more than ever. Glad everything's bought though. Joyce came and we went out for fish and chips.

27 NOVEMBER 2006

Bad night, loads of hot flushes. Used shampoo for first time since hair fell out as I've just got a slight covering now and it's very grey! Lazy day watching TV and reading. Gill came to pick me up for girlie night at my niece Suzanne's Body Shop party.

Lovely to see them all and I won the raffle prize, perhaps my luck's changing.

28 NOVEMBER 2006

Couldn't get to sleep last night and was going to have a lie in but Sally rang about coming for coffee after her Cookridge review so had to get up. Good to see her and Mike and we chatted for a couple of hours. Upset us both though I think as the last time we were out together we'd both been fit and well and dressed up for a dinner we were all invited to. After she'd gone I went upstairs and looked at the photos of us in our finery and both of us with hair and couldn't help wishing we could turn the clock back to those happier, healthy times.

29 NOVEMBER 2006

Better night. Tim's secretary rang to change next appointment time. Suzanne and Debbie picked me up and went for lunch with the girls from work. Talked about all sorts of things and really good to see them and feel included again.

30 NOVEMBER 2006

Went to see Lisa as my shoulder and chest feeling really tight after the radiotherapy so she did some massage before I saw Dr Sapsford for the cardiac ultrasound. He was lovely and in the end managed with visualisation on screen and different measurements so didn't need IV contrast. Glad about that as he explained there was a risk of reaction but probably means he'll have to be present at all the future scans for consistency or they can probably use a different measurement. Didn't fancy a bad reaction to the contrast either as I've seen patients react to other scanning drugs where they become very faint and nauseated. Anyway, the good thing is it can be sorted and I can continue on the Herceptin®.

Tips for coping with breast cancer radiotherapy
+ Daily treatments can be tiring if you drive long distances so try to get a lift from family or friends (I was lucky as we live very near Cookridge Hospital and preferred going on my own).

✦ Once the radiotherapy stops be prepared to feel a bit down as the daily trip also gives you a reason to get up and be dressed and ready on time each day. I felt pleased to complete the 15 treatments but also a bit lonely after being in company everyday.

✦ Use any skin cream as prescribed and preferably before treatment starts to prevent any sunburn-like effects. I was affected the most over the supraclavicular fossa area where I got an irritated red patch of peeling skin.

✦ Having radiotherapy can be a lonely experience and I found a little bit of conversation with the radiographers helped me to feel less isolated but equally they need to concentrate on the 'setting up' and may wish not to be distracted too much.

✦ If you have any particularly sore areas it's worth mentioning at the start of each treatment session, as I kept quiet about my hypersensitive arm until it was pulled about and really hurt during the positioning.

✦ It's preferable not to gain or lose much weight as the positioning of the tattoos may change. The radiographers had a bit of a problem with the seroma in my axilla as it changed a bit and I nearly had to have a repeat planning scan.

✦ It might be better to wear vest tops/camisoles rather than bras as the skin may become more affected as the treatment progresses.

DECEMBER: FULL OF BIRTHDAYS AND CELEBRATIONS

1 DECEMBER 2006

Phil off today. Had lie in and then went shopping and to Joyce's. It had been her friend's funeral today but she was okay afterwards. I was concerned it may bring back memories of Eric's but she seemed quite calm. Went to the Indian where my car had broken down before but this time had a nice meal with no mishaps.

2 DECEMBER 2006

My great nephew Samuel's first birthday today. Called at my parents before his party. Had chilli and jacket potato and then felt really unwell when we got home. Up to the loo to vomit six times overnight and couldn't keep count of the diarrhoea. Phil started later with the trots but not sick at all. So was it the curry or the chilli or a bug? Felt awful thinking it might be from Sam's party and hoped no one else was ill.

3 DECEMBER 2006

Awful day so weak and weary. Got up and had a bath 3.30pm but felt so awful had to lie down again. Took some Maxolon® and started to feel a bit better. Had early night, not expecting to sleep but did thankfully.

4 DECEMBER 2006

Had to get up at 9am for BUPA appointment. Phil stayed off work so knew he was still feeling bad as he's only stayed off work before when he's been hospitalised. Saw Lisa for massage and stretching my shoulder prior to having the Herceptin®. Told the IV team about the diarrhoea and vomiting and there has been a bug going round, makes sense as everyone else at Samuel's party was okay. Just drank water while the infusion was administered instead of my usual coffee and sandwiches. The 'drop dead gorgeous' boy has left, so Tracie won't want to come with me again! Eileen called and will ask Kirtida about wearing the compression sleeve again and Phil Turton about stopping wearing the chest band. Blood tests repeated today.

I was quite surprised when one of the patients started talking to me about my hair loss as I was complaining to Catherine that my eyelashes and eyebrows still wouldn't grow. I'd coincided with this girl a few times before and had always said hello but she didn't seem to want to engage at all. Today she told me how awful she'd felt about the alopecia and her loss of appetite and had become agoraphobic. It was really good to talk to her and I complimented her on her wig and how natural it looked. Made me want to help others again, so perhaps I should be thinking about returning to work but how will I ever get up in time to be in work for 8am?

5 DECEMBER 2006

Phil better, went to work and left me in bed. Didn't get up till mid-morning but felt hungry so had some cereal. Eileen rang and I can start wearing the sleeve again and hurrah – can stop wearing the band.

6 DECEMBER 2006

Awful night, hoped I would sleep better without the band but really hot and sweaty. Phil went into work early, glad to get away from me I think! I got to sleep after he'd gone and didn't wake up till 11am. Combed my hair for the first time since losing it, as I was getting ready to see Tim. Still too short without a scarf though. Think I'll see what it's like by Christmas Day for the first unveiling!

Phil picked me up in the afternoon. Tim said I was a bit neutropenic and definitely post-menopausal with my hormone levels. Asked about calcium supplements as osteoporosis prophylaxis and he thought that was a good idea along with a healthy diet and weight bearing exercises. Will need bone density scan at one year after starting the letrozole. Changed Herceptin® day to Tuesday as this will be better for me getting back to work before the year's treatment finishes in May. Talked about how I might feel being back at work and laughed about me not getting up till late everyday and how my ideal hours would be between lunchtime and 2pm! Had physio with Lisa, really hurt but better afterwards, she noticed a rash on my side and asked for Phil to keep an eye on it. Glad to get home, felt really tired.

7 DECEMBER 2006

Not as tired today but aching all over. Stayed out longer and tried to walk around a bit more. Gill called, nice to see her. Phil in a quiet mood.

8 DECEMBER 2006

Went into Leeds with Wilma and another old nursing friend Sue instead of our annual pre-Christmas shopping trip to York. I don't feel tired today but my back is aching. Think the seroma is more obvious but probably due to not wearing the strap and keeping it compressed. Wore the compression sleeve and my arm felt better, otherwise feel like I can't relax it by my side.

Got invited to friends Liz and John's Christmas party next weekend. Can't believe it's a whole year since we saw them. Phil in happier mood.

9 DECEMBER 2006

Stayed in all day and finished Christmas wrapping and cards. Phil thinks the seroma looks bigger.

10 DECEMBER 2006

Phil's uncle John's ruby anniversary and our 15th for our first date back in December 1991! The night when I knew Phil was very special. Wanted to have a really good day but started badly as Phil upset yet again that I want to see Phil Turton on my own in January. He can't accept why I like to deal with things on my own and I get sick of the ill feeling it causes and it would be solved if I just gave in and let him come with me. Tried to be more honest with him but just seem to hurt his feelings. Had to agree to disagree and went to John and Diane's party. I drove to give Phil chance to relax and enjoy a drink and I want to lose more actual weight now that the oedema has subsided. Good party, lots of champagne which I couldn't have so regretting the decision to drive!

11 DECEMBER 2006

Went to Otley. Next-door-but-one had break in last night, then when I got into Otley a car had accidentally driven into a shop front injuring the elderly couple in it. So bought Justine Picardie's book, *If the Spirit Moves You: life and love after death*, about trying to communicate with her dead sister just to cheer myself up![37] Cheered up later though, had girlie night out for Christmas at the Red Chilli and ate loads from the Chinese banquet (so much for wanting to lose weight). Catherine did the taxiing around, bless her, and it was good to see everyone.

12 DECEMBER 2006

Feel well today; hope this is the start of recovering some of the old me back.

NICE TO BE ABLE TO CUDDLE!

13 DECEMBER 2006

Wilma picked me up for physio appointment with Lisa. Told her I've been getting pins and needles in my left hand and she gave me some more stretching exercises. She thinks it might be due to the median nerve being affected from surgery. Told her how pleased I was last night in bed as managed to put my arm around Phil without it hurting for the first time in ages. Lovely flowers had been left on our doorstep when I got back home from friends JJ and Clare who I haven't seen since the diagnosis, but we've spoken on the phone and they've sent me cards to keep in touch.

14 DECEMBER 2006

Not much to say, lousy weather. Put tinsel rope over curtain rail to use as pulley system to stretch out my arm as Lisa showed me yesterday. Phil out with work so just had some soup, as I couldn't be bothered cooking for myself.

15 DECEMBER 2006

Went into work to deliver presents and cards, good to see everyone and made me feel a bit more Christmassy. Also signed form about CNS post to retain old position in light of CNS audit that's been conducted while I've been off sick. Stopped off to get some food and the drive home was awful, really busy and glad to get home safely. Forgotten what it's like to be out in the rush hour traffic.

16 DECEMBER 2006

Nice day. Mark and Keri picked us up for lunch at Bellini's. Showed them my very short grey hair and they said it suited me but perhaps they were being kind.

17 DECEMBER 2006

Up late. Decorated Christmas tree in the conservatory and put cards up. Went to Liz's party, strange seeing everyone from last year as it made me think what a difference a year makes. Good to see Russ (my old friend who's a GP), he was upset that I'd not let him know sooner. Tired standing up chatting though so didn't stay long. Arranged to meet up with Russ and his wife Alison before too long.

18 DECEMBER 2006

Wilma came and we went to the garden centres like a couple of old retirees! I feel quite ashamed to say I really enjoyed myself. Stayed at her house for a meal and Phil came over later from work.

19 DECEMBER 2006

Went to BUPA for appointment with Kirtida. Much better news as measurement okay on left so probably still settling from surgery effects rather than troublesome lymphoedema. Still to wear the compression sleeve and she showed me how to do self-lymphatic drainage as I feel my face is still puffy at times. See her in six months again and hope by then I can stop wearing the sleeve, as I'll be back at work by then. Called to see Eileen and Catherine and drop off Christmas presents.

Went to the jewellers to see if my wedding ring could be altered as it's definitely too tight now, they can stretch it but it won't be back till January. Steve rang when I got home. Joaney's suffering with painful knee ligaments so will be in a splint Christmas Day when we meet up.

20 DECEMBER 2006

Up early to meet Suzanne (my niece) at Leeds General Infirmary for her bone scan as she's been having wrist problems (seems like all the family's falling apart!). Had a quick look at the local shops while she was waiting for the isotope injection to take effect. She ran me to work when it was done and caught up with the girls in the office. Gill and Lorna came back home with me for some wine and chat.

21 DECEMBER 2006

Gill picked me up for a treat at her health club. Went for a quick swim even though it's not quite January, but all radiotherapy sites okay now as sore areas have all healed. Swimming was all right, but felt a bit of a tugging sensation in my breast as I was doing the breast stroke, so only did a couple of lengths then sat in the steam room to relax. Lovely facial as part of Gill's Christmas present to me. Felt okay without scarf in public for the first time but feel I look a bit butch with it so short.

Rang my parents when I got home and arranged to pick them up Christmas Day, but Joaney can't bend her leg at all so should be fun getting her in the car.

22 DECEMBER 2006

Set the alarm for 9am to test whether getting up earlier will help me sleep better at night. Tracie came with her daughter Carlie and we swapped presents and had a good chat. Phil home mid-afternoon for Christmas hols. Took me for GP appointment to get sick note, prescription and have the mole checked. I let Phil come in with me as he could then tell the GP about the changes on my back. She wants to refer me to a dermatologist so I asked to see Julia who's the professor I work with in the melanoma clinic. Poulam rang coincidentally and told me to ring Julia myself for early appointment, but I'll wait till I hear from her as I feel it's okay and not anything sinister.

23 DECEMBER 2006

Up earlier to take cats to the vet for their vaccinations. Showed her Suki's loss of fur on her back legs. She thinks she's been picking up the stress of what's going on with me and it's causing her to over-groom. So that's something else to feel guilty about!

Elaine and my goddaughter Anna came to swap presents. Missed seeing Elaine's other daughter Ruth as she's travelling up from London. Then Ann came and we swapped birthday presents as hers is 29th December. They all thought my hair looked good.

24 DECEMBER 2006

Had a nice lie in. Then went to church with Joyce and enjoyed singing the carols and being inside the lovely building. Felt quite nostalgic for past Christmases though, when there was less to be sad about. Or is that just normal for being an adult and losing a bit of the magic? Had a nice meal and opened most of our presents apart from Phil's and mine to each other.

25 DECEMBER 2006

Opened remaining presents in bed, just like I used to when I was a little girl. I decided today was going to be a good one with no disagreements at all. Picked up my parents and Joaney managed okay with her splint and the car journey to Steve's. Usually everyone comes to us for Christmas lunch but must admit I was glad I don't have to do it this year, as I don't feel I would have the energy for all the preparation. Lovely family day (from one-year-old Samuel to the oldies in their eighties), everyone liked my hair and I just ate and drank and opened presents! Felt tired but good to be with everyone.

26 DECEMBER 2006

Up early for the Rhinos rugby match with Wakefield. Went with friends and enjoyed being out in the fresh air. Got bad backache while standing, but the whisky in the hip flask helped! Joyce had made us a lovely meal when we got back. Packed for my birthday trip, as we have to be at BUPA early in the morning.

27 DECEMBER 2006

Finished packing and got to BUPA early for Herceptin®. Cannula painful throughout infusion, but it infused okay. Stopped off for lunch before we arrived at the Traddock in Austwick. It's a lovely old country house hotel and very Christmassy with the open fires and candlelight. Opened some birthday presents and had delicious meal. Couldn't sleep.

I'VE BEEN HERE FOR HALF A CENTURY!

28 DECEMBER 2006

Can't believe I'm 50 years old today, although I've felt more like 90 at times recently. Took my cards down to the elegant breakfast room with piped classical music and had a laugh as Mark and Keri's card played disco music when I opened it and surprised the other guests. Not great weather but didn't stop us enjoying a walk to Clapham and back. Stopped at the pub halfway round and was glad of the rest, but also had a blister from my new boots. Feel very fat today, but decided to enjoy the evening meal again and worry about weight later. Slept a bit better.

29 DECEMBER 2006

Left for home by 11am. Arm aching so put the compression sleeve on and interestingly Phil commented how I don't move it as much as I did before when I'm walking. Hadn't realised that myself but makes sense as to why it feels stiff and aching. Rang my parents when we got home. They've got colds so not to call as we were planning tomorrow. Joaney had fluid drained from her knee and splint now removed.

Went to friends Di and Reg's wedding party at night and really good to see everyone. Got more presents from friends I haven't seen in a while. Great live band, but Phil very quiet and wouldn't dance. Decided to ignore his mood and make the most of the party.

30 DECEMBER 2006

Fell out a bit over last night. Told Phil about living life to the full, which I think I always have done, and want to continue doing. Feel he misses out when he won't join in and let his hair down. Better mood by the time we set off to Elaine's, but then things got worse than ever. Lovely to see my goddaughter Ruth who was home from London, but then we started talking about Elaine's new job at Wakefield Hospice. I went into 'work mode' and we were talking about palliative care issues she might have to face as a psychologist. I was aware that Phil got up and went into the other room but he didn't say anything to us. He had thought he was starting with a cold so assumed he wasn't feeling too well. When I saw him though, I knew he was upset again, so we left early. In the car, on the way home he told me he was very upset and I shouldn't have carried on talking to Elaine. Couldn't be bothered talking to him as he seems to be getting upset whenever we are in friends' company and didn't want to argue while he was driving. I did ask him why he hadn't said our conversation was upsetting him, as Elaine would definitely have understood and we would have changed the subject.

31 DECEMBER 2006

Phil apologised and I decided to try and be a bit more under-standing, but asked him to just be honest if we're out and not stay quiet if he's upset at the time. Don't want to keep feeling like I'm 'treading on eggshells' and hoped we'd sorted out our differences. So glad to feel closer again as I've said many times this past few months. Gill and Alistair due to come over for a meal but Gill rang to cancel as Al's too busy on call. Probably a good thing to be on our own as Phil's cold worse, but was very touched as he asked to speak to Gill and thanked her for all she'd done for me this past year. Turned into a good New Year's Eve as we watched *Narnia* and *Monsters Inc.* Toasted in 2007 with Lemsip® and went to bed straight after midnight, glad that 2006 is over!

A NEW YEAR: IS IT GOING TO BE A GOOD ONE?

1 JANUARY 2007

Over to my niece Caroline's via my parents for a Greek meal and another birthday present as she had forgotten to bring it for me on Christmas Day. Left early though as Phil not well with his cold, but I didn't mind as he'd made a big effort to join in the chat with all my family while we were there.

2 JANUARY 2007

Went to Harrogate for the sales and enjoyed being out walking. My joints are really sore and struggled with bags back to the car.
    Phil's old friend Gary rang and he explained what had been happening to me, as I'd let Gary and his wife Kay know via their

Christmas card. Phil was concerned about whether he'd described things accurately and appropriately, and it made me sorry for the times I've dismissed his feelings, as I forget he doesn't have the same medical knowledge as most of my friends. I'm sure this is why we have conflict, as we're very comfortable discussing cancer and palliative care issues in our 'work mode', and of course it's all very emotional for Phil at the moment.

3 JANUARY 2007

Not much to say, nice not to think too much for a change.

4 JANUARY 2007

Out to the dentist, and pleased he thinks my teeth are okay. Thought they might have suffered a bit with the chemo.

Reflection

I've recently had to have some white filling in my front teeth as the enamel was eroding. The dentist was a bit puzzled why and asked me if I've been eating lots of fruit. I do eat loads again since my taste returned to normal. He reminded me about not brushing my teeth straight after drinking fruit juice or eating fruit, as the acid from the fruit can be brushed into the tooth enamel. He also prescribed some fluoride fortified toothpaste. Perhaps I should stick with the chocolate and chips!

5 JANUARY 2007

Up early to see Phil Turton. He was pleased with how I looked, took more photos and talked about nipple reconstruction under local anaesthetic. But I wanted to have a mastopexy done on the other side at the same time if possible. I just feel if I'm more symmetrical in shape it will help me to feel better about my body again. Phil Turton also thinks it will be a good cosmetic result as I haven't got huge boobs! He'll write to the insurers and explained I'd be in for two nights and need about two weeks recovery. I'm sure it'll be worth it to make me feel balanced and complete again. Told him about trying to get this done before I go back to work. Also offered to remove the mole at the same time. Did consider asking for an 'eye job' too but that might be going too far! Called to see Catherine and had a nice chat about future plans. Tried Kalms® again to get to sleep.

6 JANUARY 2007

Went to the pantomime at York – *Cinderella* (Mark and Keri's birthday present to me). Their three grown up kids came with us and we had a really good night shouting 'he's behind you!', and booing and hissing at the 'baddies'.

7 JANUARY 2007

Lovely day with Phil, just enjoyed being together.

8 JANUARY 2007

Went for a swim, first time back at the Parkway Hotel since surgery, etc. Enjoyed being back in the water and felt like I'd quite a bit of energy. Felt really fat in my new swimming costume though. Glad I bought this one with a built in bra and higher neck and sides as feel my armpit needs more coverage now. Some of the other members made comments at not seeing me for a while. One lady said I'd put on weight then got embarrassed when I said I hadn't been able to exercise for a while. She apologised as she remembered I'd been ill and changed her opinion to 'You look blooming'.

9 JANUARY 2007

Couldn't be bothered writing anything till the 15th so can't remember much of what happened. Still feel compelled to record something everyday though as I'm worried I'll miss something significant.

10 JANUARY 2007

Wilma picked me up and went over to my parents. Had nice lunch in the café but remember it was very windy and cold for them walking. Phil out at a meeting in the evening but called home for ten minutes to see me briefly before he left. Long evening without him.

11 JANUARY 2007

Went to the jewellers for my wedding ring, but it's not ready yet. Hate being without it even though I'm wearing another ring in its place. It belonged to Joyce before me, as Phil's father bought it for her when they got married, so I feel it's very sentimental for Phil. His father died when he was a very small baby so he doesn't have any memories of him. Called for a swim on the way home.

12 JANUARY 2007

Went to the chemist for owed letrozole tablets again. Then for a swim. Saw one of the men who swims regularly and he'd seen me before, when I was wearing my bandana. Today he said, 'Oh I didn't know they still shaved your head when you went to prison'. I was a bit stunned, so just laughed and got out of the pool to sit in the steam room. Just when I was beginning to gain my confidence back and stop wearing a scarf. I couldn't help but feel angry with him, even though I realise it was just a throwaway comment. Made me think of all the patients going through the same process and how a knock back can affect us. Told Phil in the evening and was pleased he was angry about it rather than dismissing it as a funny comment.

13 JANUARY 2007

Busy day, cleaning and sorting out spare bedroom. Went to a local restaurant at night for Phil's colleague's retirement party. Ate late though, and not very enjoyable sorting drinks bill out. I wanted to get everyone organised, and for once Phil wanted to sit back and relax.

14 JANUARY 2007

Our 12th wedding anniversary. Went to Joyce's for a meal and I was going to drive but my arm was aching so much, Phil took over. Couldn't help but reminisce about how I looked in our wedding day photo that Joyce keeps on her mantelpiece in comparison to today.

15 JANUARY 2007

Went to aqua aerobics and felt good afterwards. Debbie came for a coffee and brought cake. Had a good chat and she thought my hair and eyebrows had grown. I'm still not hopeful about my eyebrows and eyelashes returning fully as it seems to be taking so long. Also noticed my finger ends more numb than ever today. Phil very tired when he got home as he had had a bad day at work.

16 JANUARY 2007

Up early for BUPA appointment. 12th Herceptin® today so only five more to go for the full year's treatment. Catherine away on holiday so mentioned my finger numbness to Jane as she was cannulating me and she said it might last a whole year. Bit of retail therapy afterwards and booked a facial.

17 JANUARY 2007

Up to go to work to park and get the shuttle bus to Seacroft Hospital for mole check. Called in to see the palliative care team and had a good chat with Dawn who's been so good to me with advice and regular phone calls. Went over to outpatients at Seacroft to see Julia about the mole. It's just aging (like me!) and not a problem but she thought it would be a good idea to have it removed by Phil Turton at the same time as my next operation. Nice to see the girls in the office when I got back to St James's.

18 JANUARY 2007

Awful windy day today. Went to aqua aerobics to try and help my aches and pains.

19 JANUARY 2007

Went to the jewellers again and glad to get my wedding ring back. Bought valerian tablets to try and aid sleep. Got Isle of Man brochures to try and get a holiday sorted for later this year. Had a nice evening, as Phil seems much happier again.

20 JANUARY 2007

Lie in with Phil. Nice day apart from my nails are sore and seem to be lifting off again on my left hand, just when I thought they were growing okay. Joyce came for a meal.

21 JANUARY 2007

Really good day. Went over to Sheffield and lovely to see our friends Ruth and Tony and godchildren. Finally swapped Christmas presents but the kids enjoyed getting them late. Had to leave earlier than planned though as it started snowing quite heavily.

22 JANUARY 2007

Nice lie in but also felt I slept better last night. Went to aqua aerobics and enjoyed the exercise. Spoke to my friend Sue about returning to work, she thought I might not want to stay in nursing. Surprised how many people think I should still give it up.

23 JANUARY 2007

Had lovely, relaxing facial today and nice to get neck and shoulder massage. Really miss the regular massages I used to have on my back, neck and shoulders but wouldn't enjoy it the same as my back is still overly sensitive in some areas.

24 JANUARY 2007

Went swimming and not much else to say. It's actually quite good not to have anything dramatic going on. I'd settle for a boring life for a while.

25 JANUARY 2007

Enjoyed aqua aerobics. Walked to Bellini's for a meal with Gill and Alistair. Really good evening and we shared a taxi back home. Then couldn't sleep.

26 JANUARY 2007

Phil up really early. I had lie in and went swimming. Went to Rhinos rugby match at Headingley in the evening and it was a really good testimonial match. Glad to get back to the car though.

Phil very considerate and was going to park nearer the ground, but I think I need to push myself a bit more to improve my stamina.

27 JANUARY 2007

Went to the supermarket to stock up for family meal tomorrow and bumped into Poulam again. Shopping on his own this time. Had really good chat and blocked the vegetable aisle with our trolleys for ages annoying quite a few people around us! Watched the film *The Green Mile* in the evening and cried and cried.

28 JANUARY 2007

Family came and we had a nice evening, but then fell out with Phil as he was doing all the clearing up as usual and I wanted him to sit and relax with us all.

29 JANUARY 2007

Up early to see Kath who's taken over from the previous oncology matron Angela. We had a good meeting, she was very fair and we discussed dates for a phased return. Told her I was waiting for a date for surgery and will let her know as soon as it's confirmed at BUPA. Also saw a patient who I treated with chemotherapy years ago who's had multiple surgery and is waiting for a brain operation. Made me feel really guilty and pathetic for worrying about my nails and hair, etc.

30 JANUARY 2007

Drove over to my parents, first time on my own for a long time. Their GP was there when I arrived as Joaney's leg pain bad again. Went into Ossett just with Pop to get her prescription but very windy and he nearly fell over. Feel guilty for neglecting them this past year but honestly couldn't have driven over before today and I know they understand. We've tried to stay close by sending cards and talking on the phone but I've really missed being with them.

31 JANUARY 2007

Wilma came over and we went to see Joyce. She's been brilliant during all my time off work. Phil rang trying to sort out holiday insurance for me for June 2007 if we go to the Isle of Man as the quotes are all really expensive. The premium is high as I won't be six months post-treatment, as the Herceptin®, surgery and letrozole are ongoing. Tried through Help the Aged who are kinder about a cancer diagnosis and they've suggested Free Spirit insurers (www.free-spirit.com).

1 FEBRUARY 2007

Went to aqua aerobics and then did some packing for our annual London weekend trip (dinner/dance for Phil's company at the Berkeley Hotel).

2 FEBRUARY 2007

Phil really upset after speaking to Joyce, her friend Rita died last night with breast cancer recurrence. He'd known her all his life, as they were neighbours when he was a baby. Didn't have the courage to ask him if he was more upset because she died of breast cancer.

Went by train to London. Good location hotel right opposite to Harrods. Enjoyed the afternoon just at the local shops, especially Harrods' food hall. Italian meal at night and felt okay seeing everyone although it's a year since I saw most of them. They were all very positive about my short hair. Couldn't sleep despite valerian tablets and feeling really tired.

3 FEBRUARY 2007

Met up for breakfast and I had the healthy option while all the others tucked into a 'full English'. We all went our separate ways and we walked to the river and had a quick look in Harvey Nicks before Phil went to the pub to watch the rugby. I just rested on the bed in the hotel, annoyed that I didn't have the energy to do anything else. We walked to the Berkeley Hotel in the evening, lovely meal and had a few dances with Phil. Didn't have the stamina to stay till the end though so we walked back on our own. Felt a bit sad thinking about previous years when we'd have been amongst the last to leave and certainly the last on the dance floor.

4 FEBRUARY 2007

Breakfast in the room and then left early for the train. Reserved seats were facing backwards which I hate as it makes me nauseated. The carriage was so warm and packed I had to wait by the doors till it set off. Felt okay though once I sat down, as I concentrated on reading the entire journey rather than looking at the scenery. Loads of people had to stand, at least we had a seat. Glad to get home, loads of calls on answer machine, including invites from friends for meals.

IS TALKING GOOD EXERCISE?

5 FEBRUARY 2007

Went to aqua aerobics, and then met my friend Alison at Bellini's for lunch. Really good to see her and had long chat. We were the last in the restaurant and then carried on talking in the car park as all the staff were leaving for home. Out again in the evening to Dean and Tracie's for a home-cooked meal. Felt really tired on the way home despite having all my meals made for me today, perhaps it was all the talking!

6 FEBRUARY 2007

Herceptin® again today, had another good chat with Catherine and grateful she's so good at cannulating as my right hand veins are getting a bit worn out. The Herceptin® seems to be making me more tired now and I was glad to get home. Had to force myself to stay awake. Hope this isn't an accumulation of the cardiac effects as I hope to complete the full year's course. Even though my heart hasn't been adversely affected on the regular ultrasound scans, I feel the Herceptin® slows me down and definitely has an effect on my energy level.

7 FEBRUARY 2007

Enjoyed a lie in. Went for a swim but feel lonely today despite being with other people.

8 FEBRUARY 2007

Better day, Wilma came and we did the aqua aerobics together and had a nice lunch. Phil rang about sorting BUPA insurance codes for next operation and insurance for holidays. So glad he's sorting all the administration stuff, I haven't got the patience he has. We talked about me going to Rita's funeral with him, but I felt I would get too upset and emotional and that would be inappropriate because I didn't know her. I would be upset for him and Joyce, and for myself for the threat that breast cancer holds for my future. My ribs are really hurting today; hope I haven't overdone the exercising.

9 FEBRUARY 2007

Went shopping and had hassle as checkout broke down and I was tired and joints aching but once fixed the cashier helped me pack. Phil had been home to change for the funeral. Felt guilty for not going with him but think it was the right decision. I would have been very emotional at just being in the church as it's also just three years tomorrow since his stepfather, Eric, died as well as thinking about the breast cancer connection. Started snowing really heavily so glad when Phil got home safely. We cancelled meeting up with old friends Gary and Kay, as the snow got worse during the early evening. Shame though, as we haven't seen them for ages and they're going skiing tomorrow with their three girls, so won't be able to rearrange for a while.

10 FEBRUARY 2007

Lazy day, feel a bit down and not just because of Eric's anniversary. Keep wondering about our future as I've always worried about Phil's health and now I'm wondering about mine too. Met up with Joyce for a meal at Bellini's, as she wanted to treat us and her neighbours who've been very kind to her since Eric's death. We toasted Eric and I tried to join in the conversation but felt a bit strange and remote from it all. I couldn't really enjoy being there without him as he was the 'life and soul' of any gathering and life's been a lot quieter without him.

11 FEBRUARY 2007

Nice day with Phil. Tried to be a bit happier today and not so introspective.

12 FEBRUARY 2007

Bad night and disturbed Phil so he got up early. Ribs really hurting so good to be able to stretch out once he got up. Wondering whether I ought to go back to the spare room, as I don't want to keep disturbing his sleep, but the number of hot sweats and my joint discomfort is no better. Went to GP with letter for a sick note and repeat prescription on the way to aqua aerobics.

13 FEBRUARY 2007

Decided to stay out a bit longer today as a test for returning to work so went shopping and then swimming. Tried to walk a bit more, parked at the top of the street and not too breathless getting back to the car. Pleased, as it's uphill.

14 FEBRUARY 2007

Valentine's Day, lovely card from Phil. Hope he still loves me like before. Went swimming and for a walk round the lake in the park. Lovely sunny day and all the spring flowers are beginning to surface. Made a nice meal and enjoyed pink champagne when Phil got home.

15 FEBRUARY 2007

Went to aqua aerobics, can't remember much else but not as exciting as yesterday. No more pink champagne!

16 FEBRUARY 2007

Picked up sick note and prescription from GP. Shopped and glad to get home, as feel tired and out at Debbie's tonight. Went to her Body Shop party and good to see the girls from work. All positive comments about my hair, as this is the first time some of them have seen me without a scarf and they all think I look well.

17 FEBRUARY 2007

Good day. Went to Bellini's with all the family for Pop's eighty-third birthday and he paid for us all. Fourteen month old Samuel kept us amused, as he now says 'hiya' to everyone. Came back to us for drinks and lovely to be with everyone, but my brother Steve not too happy as he's waiting for cardiac test results.

18 FEBRUARY 2007

Rang Pop to wish him happy birthday and he really enjoyed last night too. Busy day then cleaning up and sorting out. Feel a bit more energetic today.

19 FEBRUARY 2007

Aqua aerobics session good but ribs hurting on the left side again. Phil Turton's secretary rang, still waiting for insurance decision for next operation. Rang Steve as he was seeing the cardiologist about results of his stress test. Possibly is getting angina or could be hypertension causing his chest pain. Given different medication and will be seen in three months again. He's only in his fifties so hope this isn't serious.

20 FEBRUARY 2007

Up earlier to take sick note into work and see the girls in the office. Met Wilma in Leeds and had good look around. Pretty tired by the time I got home and worried about my stamina for being back at work in April. Phil out for business meal. Good news when he came home as he's been speaking to the BUPA insurers and Phil Turton's secretary. We may still have to pay some of the cost afterwards but can go ahead as planned on 2nd March without having to pay anything beforehand. I hope it will be covered because I wouldn't choose this surgery unless I felt it completely necessary to finish off my treatment and return from an ill person to a healthy one. I feel without this final bit I will always be looking in the mirror and seeing the difference in breast shape and nipple position. Particularly since the hormone changes and droopiness. It's bad enough only having one nipple but I would prefer it to be central and not heading south! Phil Turton's explained to me that he makes a cut under the breast and up to and around the nipple area. These usually heal very well and fade with time.

<u>21 FEBRUARY 2007</u>

Was going to get up earlier again but couldn't get out of bed. So many hot sweats that I can't sleep for long and having trouble getting to sleep despite taking valerian. Went to Otley for a walk around and called at Joyce's. Stopped off for a swim.

NO EYEBROWS OR EYELASHES BUT I'VE GOT TWO CHINS!

<u>22 FEBRUARY 2007</u>

Poor night again but got up for aqua aerobics and felt better after exercise. Spoke to a new lady and she didn't realise I'd been ill, as we continued speaking and when I mentioned I'd had a long break from work she assumed it was my choice. Made me feel more confident about my appearance as when I look in the mirror I still see no eyebrows, small piggy eyes with no eyelashes and a double chin! Eileen rang from BUPA, as we've not spoken for a while. Talked about admission on 2nd March and appointment for ultrasound so she'll see me later. Got pre-assessment forms through the post so will take them in later. Cardiac ultrasound okay, still uncomfortable though with pressure on my ribs, guess this is a side effect of the radiotherapy as I know it can cause discomfort for quite a time afterwards. Saw Eileen and gave her pre-op forms. First time she's seen my hair and she thought I looked good. Glad to get home as feeling tired.

<u>23 FEBRUARY 2007</u>

Stopped vitamin E today as I remembered Phil Turton advised that before the last surgery. Not looking forward to possible increase in flushes and night sweats as a result of stopping the capsules. Phil home today for our weekend away with Mark and Keri. Set off late morning for Austwick and had a good journey. I felt a bit strange though as couldn't help reflecting on our trip a year ago and how I've nearly gone 'full circle' from suspicion of malignancy to nearing completion of treatment. Also remembering how I had to be falsely cheerful with everyone last year despite knowing I had a potential problem to get sorted on going home. Had a good laugh with Phil at the pub he chose for lunch, as when we got inside there was no other customers, no windows, no fire and the landlord said they weren't doing food! Had a swift half pint of beer and went to the pub near our guesthouse instead. Lovely place to stay. Our room was really good with beams and great view. Mark and Keri arrived late afternoon and, as always with them, we had a really good evening.

24 FEBRUARY 2007

No sleep, watched the clock all night and got really upset at 3am, nearly got up to sit downstairs. Great breakfast and despite the awful weather we had a really good day. Walked to the same pub as yesterday but much better today as the fire was lit and lots of people coming in to get dry. We took turns to stand in front of the fire and had a good banter with other walkers and cyclists. Still no food though so ate loads of crisps instead! Glad I could do the walk but couldn't keep up with the others and had to stop several times when going uphill. Had a lie down when we got back while Phil watched the rugby with Mark. Lovely meal at night at the Traddock Hotel where we went for my birthday.

25 FEBRUARY 2007

Better night. Walked again, just four miles or so but far enough as I found it really tiring climbing over all the stiles. Really funny sensation when I pull up with my left arm, as I can feel the muscle in my breast moving and it feels weird. Nice meal at the pub with Mark and Keri before they left early evening. Seemed very quiet once they'd gone, as we were the only guests for Sunday night. Read about Justine Picardie's sister Ruth again in the Sunday papers and it made me feel sad, as she was so young and only lived for 11 months after diagnosis. I could readily identify with a lot of her sentiments such as retail therapy being rather more effective than chemotherapy and much more fun![38]

26 FEBRUARY 2007

Home via Joyce's. Phil's auntie and uncle were there so nice to see them. Uncle John needs radiotherapy now for prostate cancer so we talked a bit about his consultant, as I know her. I tried to reassure him about how much support he will get during the treatment and how he should ask if he's unsure or worried about anything as he has a tendency to faint every time he has a hospital visit and he has to have 20 sessions of radiotherapy.

I went for a swim in the afternoon and sat in the steam room to get rid of my muscle stiffness from the walking. Spoke to my parents and they were pleased to hear from me but sad for John.

27 FEBRUARY 2007

Another Herceptin® day. Had bloods done too which will be good for pre-theatre check to ensure I'm fit for anaesthetic and surgery. Glad to get home, particularly with going back tomorrow to see Tim. Phil commented about me disturbing his sleep. I think the night sweats are worse with stopping the vitamin E.

28 FEBRUARY 2007

Slept okay, but made up the spare bed again as I have to lie so still to not wake Phil that I then get more joint pains. Saw Tim early afternoon and told him about the persisting flushes and sweats. He's recommended venlaflaxine and will write to my GP for it to be prescribed. Tim told me Tuesday's bloods were all okay and my female hormone levels remain rock bottom so he wasn't surprised about the flushes, etc. as I'm truly menopausal. He wasn't going to examine me in view of surgery on Friday but I told him about noticing a prominent vein on my chest again and so he checked me over and it's nothing to worry about. I was just a bit concerned in case it was increased blood supply to another suspicious area. Felt a bit foolish and aware I'm probably noticing more, as I probably look at my chest a lot more than I used to. Also felt embarrassed, as I was very flushed and hot and worried about my sweaty armpits.

Tim suggested I have a yearly mammogram on the right breast and it's due in mid-March. But I managed to get one done before

I left, otherwise I would have had to wait a few months post-surgery for any soreness to settle. Feel sure the result will be okay but couldn't help wondering if it isn't clear and if there isn't time to report it before I'm being operated on will that spread things around? If there are any cancer cells present in the right side where the calcification was and Phil Turton goes ahead with surgery before a report of the mammogram is available, then that could be bad news. I can only hope that my hunch is correct and there's no problem. Went for a swim before home. Slept in the spare room, as I wanted to stretch out and felt much cooler in there.

1 MARCH 2007

Went to aqua aerobics and enjoyed exercising quite vigorously. Packed for the ward and debating where to sleep as I would like to be with Phil but definitely more comfortable on my own. When Phil came home we didn't talk much as he seemed quite agitated and I didn't want to argue. Decided to sleep in the spare room and set the alarm for 7.30 as I've to fast from 8am tomorrow morning.

MORE BAD NEWS AS 'FINISHING OFF' OPERATION CANCELLED

2 MARCH 2007

Didn't sleep well, but expected that. Got up to make myself some coffee and cereal and Keri rang to wish me luck and joked about not coming back with 'Jordan' breasts. Phil still quiet but nice that he's with me today. He answered the phone to Dr Chapman ringing from St James's. I was just about to get in the bath in preparation for BUPA when he changed the plans. He'd had a look at the mammogram and compared it to the first one twelve months ago. He didn't want to alarm me but the area of calcification has increased in size and apparently this is quite unusual. So my 'hunch' was incorrect and the problems I was worried about with the mammogram showing a problem area have happened. Thankfully Dr Chapman was able to check the pictures but he didn't know I was due in for surgery and thought this should be postponed. He promised to ring Phil Turton to discuss it further.

He told me it could be new DCIS or more benign calcification and I would need another stereotactic biopsy. He rang me back after speaking to Phil Turton and so no surgery today and I will have to go to St James's on Monday for the biopsy.

Phil Turton rang me as well which I really appreciated and we talked about how I thought the op today was going to be the finish of things for my body image. He spoke frankly about the mammogram and suggested I prepare for this being new DCIS and that the best outcome may be another mastectomy. He thinks I may just have genetically bad breast tissue and even if this proves to be benign again it just means future worry looking for changes. So I was probably born with a pre-disposition to breast cancer whatever I did with my life and habits, etc. The website for breastcancer.org reports on a study of 745 women undergoing contralateral mastectomy and concludes that women may benefit from surgery if they have a family breast cancer history as well. So I'll take comfort in the fact that I'm a 'one off' in my family and my level of risk of developing a new cancer in the right side is not too bad (www.breastcancer.org).[39]

My Phil hates the idea of me going through more major surgery but equally thinks it would be preferable to the threat. I rang Gill and she told me about the need for surgery only, as if it is DCIS, it doesn't need follow-up chemotherapy or radiotherapy as it can all be removed at surgery, so at least that was good news. She offered to go with me on Monday so I'm going to meet her in our office. I then rang Steve to ask him to let my parents know the change in plan and reason for it, I felt awful telling him as I always rely on him to pass on my bad news to them.

Phil rang BUPA to sort out the biopsy procedure codes again and didn't have a very efficient response, so I rang Belinda at St James's to ask for advice and told her about the latest develop-ments as it's ages since we spoke. Eventually got through to the private patients' prices person but it was her voicemail and by then I just lost patience and said to Phil 'let's just get out of here'. We went for a walk through the woods and to the pub, which helped to calm us both, and I explained a bit more to Phil about potential treatments. We discussed me having another mastectomy and he's in favour of this to exclude any more cancer threat in the future. I'm not so sure about such drastic surgery and need to talk to Phil Turton to understand his reasoning. Also explained how even if the area is bigger it will still be contained if it's the calcification so that means chemo or radiotherapy isn't necessary. It was lovely to be out in the fresh air and clear our heads a bit. I moved back into our room, as I didn't want to be on my own overnight.

3 MARCH 2007

Went out to the café and supermarket but I didn't enjoy being in there with all the other people and was glad to get home. Feeling a bit angrier today, as I thought I had a plan for returning to work and putting all this behind me by May. Also thinking about the holidays we've got planned again and don't want them to be affected like last year. Still I know the choices will become clearer after the biopsy result so will just have to wait. Phil Turton hoped to get a result for the MDT Tuesday morning and promised to ring me as soon as he could next week.

I decided in the evening that if I have to have another mastectomy and Phil Turton can do the skin-sparing method again then I wouldn't need to have any nipple reconstruction if the result is as good as my left side. Talked to my Phil about it and he agrees entirely as he says he doesn't really see a difference now. I feel very lucky that he's so understanding, it must be terrible for women who can't show their new bodies to their partners for fear of rejection.

4 MARCH 2007

Joyce called with some flowers for me but didn't stay long as we were going to see the Rhinos. Lousy weather, raining, windy and cold so I got a bit tetchy with Phil as if it was his fault! Had a bit of walking about the ground and waiting in long queues for the tickets and I just got fed up with it all. I hope he knows me well enough to realise it's the situation I'm cross with and that anything not going to plan always upsets me. Had a nice meal in the Chinese afterwards and I felt calmer in the evening. Strangely I think Phil does too as he admits he felt very apprehensive about me having the mastopexy as he saw that as purely cosmetic surgery to give me an uplift on the right side. However, if I have to have another mastectomy to remove the right breast for more cancer he knows that's a necessary operation and can deal with it as he did the left side.

5 MARCH 2007

Went to aqua aerobics and explained to the ladies about the need for the biopsy later so they were very supportive. I went to St James's early and into the office as I didn't want to be on my own and talked to Gill and the girls before going over to the Breast Unit. I had the stereotactic biopsy done successfully as Dr Chapman got four good core specimens. The radiographer tried to just use ultrasound but the area didn't show up enough for him to target the calcification so had to use the x-ray machine. She told me not to expect a result before the end of the week. I was glad to get home and took some paracetamol, as the area feels quite sore. Eileen had left a message while I was out so rang her at BUPA and had a long chat.

6 MARCH 2007

Strange day, waiting for the 'verdict'. I stayed in and had loads of phone calls from family and friends. My niece Suzanne is pregnant again so that was lovely news and just found out that Gill's expecting too.

Each time the phone rang I wondered if it was Phil Turton as he hoped to get a result today. Thankfully he rang early evening and it's more benign calcification so we can go back to the original plan for the mastopexy and he can excise the affected area at the same time. It's about the size of a plum that needs cutting out. He told me to 'crack open the champagne' and although I'm delighted not to have more malignancy I feel like I've lots of unanswered questions about the implications of leaving the breast tissue in situ. I can't help wondering if I will always have to worry about the right side becoming malignant as well. My Phil feels the same so will be glad to get to the appointment with Phil Turton on 12th March. Checked my records and it was the 14th March 2006 when I was told about the first biopsy result from the right breast. Is it going to be like this each time I have a mammogram? I know that's the concern for my Phil and he said he really didn't know what we were celebrating as he feels a bit confused.

7 MARCH 2007

Lovely sunny day so I went out shopping and for a swim. Lovely bunch of flowers on the doorstep from Ann when I got home. I feel happier today and more settled about things again. Obviously I didn't want to have to face another mastectomy so it'll be really good if Phil Turton can allay our fears of future problems. Perhaps it's time for me to ask a few statistics about DCIS, etc. at the next appointment. Glad to see Phil as he was out in the evening for a business meal so didn't get home till late. Wilma rang so told her about the traumatic few days.

8 MARCH 2007

Nice day again, sunny and bright. Rang the GP to check about Tim's letter for the prescription and had to get his secretary to fax them a copy even though she posted it to them on Monday. They will have a prescription ready in the morning. Went to aqua aerobics and then to the café and sat outside with the sun on my face. Did the supermarket shopping and then hurt my shoulder and left arm as the trolley nearly tipped over in the car park and I grabbed it without thinking.

9 MARCH 2007

Lovely day with Wilma as she took me to the GPs for the venla-faxine prescription and I picked it up from the chemist before going to Fountain's Abbey for a walk round the grounds and two visits to the café. I'll really miss our trips out when she starts her new job. I couldn't have driven as my shoulder still hurts from yesterday.

10 MARCH 2007

Went over to Joaney and Pop's. They were really pleased to see me and I got an extra big hug from them both. Took Mother's Day present for Joaney and promised to let them know the new plan after I've seen Phil Turton on 12th March.

11 MARCH 2007

Nice day so tidied up our garden pond and did a bit of weeding around the spring flowers. Joyce came for a meal and I gave her her Mother's Day present, as we won't see her next Sunday.

12 MARCH 2007

Went to aqua aerobics and then back home before the afternoon appointment with Phil Turton. Feel a bit tense about it but not sure why. I think it's because I need to confront my future risks and I've tried not to ask about this officially. My Phil picked me up as I think he too needs to listen to the new plan and reasoning behind it. As always, Phil Turton was lovely. He explained how the calcification was confined to one area and not spread all over as I had thought from seeing the screen during the stereotactic biopsy. I was forgetting that the area that I could see was magnified, so I thought it was a much larger area that was involved. Sometimes having a bit of medical knowledge is a hindrance as a patient, as it's easy to jump to the wrong conclusions. He wants to remove the tissue around it, which will be approximately the size of a plum and can fill the space with the breast tissue he's uplifting during the mastopexy. He did mention me being in the poor prognostic group to start with but how I'd moved into the good by getting such a good response with the primary chemotherapy. We also talked about prophylactic mastectomy and I'm pleased I can retain my breast, as there isn't either a medical need or psychological need on my part to have it removed. I've decided I'm not going to constantly worry about the breast cancer returning in the right side. That would just be a waste of my life and I now feel reassured after Phil Turton's explanations today (I later read a good paper explaining more about this in further detail).[40]

Phil Turton gave me the option of surgery on 17th March, but we'd planned a weekend away for my Phil's birthday so will postpone till nearer Easter.

We went for a Thai meal before going home and Phil knew I was mulling over things. I told him how scared I'd been last year at the diagnosis and yet when you're going through all the treatment phases the fear goes away a bit as you're occupied with the interventions and get such good support from the oncology teams. He talked about when he had the auto-transplant and how he hadn't realised the seriousness of his situation until afterwards.

13 MARCH 2007

I slept a bit better and not sure if it's the venlafaxine or a placebo effect but although still hot flushes not having the drenching sweats. Went for a swim and then met Wilma for our last 'ladies who lunch' as she starts work again next week. Also had a lovely relaxing facial and scalp massage. Spoke to Kath, the oncology matron, and she was very understanding about the surgery date changing my 'back to work' plan. So will need to get another sick note for April and then do a 'phased return' through May, which will give me more time to get over the Herceptin® effects too.

14 MARCH 2007

Awful day as Phil woke me to say my MOT was due and both of us had forgotten it. Managed to get my car booked in at the garage but they couldn't do it till early afternoon so walked home – about five miles, no buses and didn't have enough cash for a taxi. I was really exhausted when I got home. Luckily the car passed the MOT and Phil gave me a lift to pick it up and then went back to work.

A WHOLE YEAR SINCE I WORKED

15 MARCH 2007

A year since I gave up work, so I feel a bit strange today. Thought I'd be well over all the treatment by now, and I still have to complete the Herceptin® and surgery. Went to aqua aerobics and then to Harrogate. Really pleased as I managed to get the Bob Seger CD that Phil wants for his birthday. Felt really tired walking back to the car and had to sit down on the benches on the Stray. The crocuses looked lovely and it feels so good that spring is arriving again.

16 MARCH 2007

Phil off work today for our Middleham trip instead of a work's Christmas party. Phil's department wanted to go walking in the Dales. Lovely guesthouse full of antiques and we had great food. Had a lazy afternoon and then met Phil's colleague Brian and his wife Claudia for a delicious meal and really enjoyed their company.

17 MARCH 2007

Phil's birthday, so glad I'm not going into BUPA Hospital today, as I would have felt so guilty for spoiling our plans. Woke early and got up to see all the horses being taken onto the moor for their training. Didn't need an alarm clock with the sound of all the hooves going past at 7am. Met the rest of Phil's work group and had a six mile walk with a good stay at the pub at four miles. Lovely evening meal with everyone.

18 MARCH 2007

Snowing today for our journey back, and much colder. Spoke to Joaney and Joyce for Mother's Day. This day always makes me feel a bit sad as I'll never be a mother, but I'm very lucky to have my lovely nieces and godchildren.

19 MARCH 2007

Slept better than in a long time, but still needed a lie in before aqua aerobics. Decided I'm going to stop writing every day now as I don't feel the same need to document how I'm feeling. But will continue till 21st March which will be a full year since my first chemotherapy and I'd like to record the effects I'm still recovering from.

20 MARCH 2007

Herceptin® again today. Had to run my hand under the hot water as it's a very cold day today and my veins were hiding. Checked with Catherine about taking vitamin E as well as venlaflaxine and that's fine so will restart it later. Did some shopping then went home, as I didn't have any energy for swimming.

A very cold but sunny day, so went into Golden Acre Park and walked round the lake to see the spring flowers. Loads of daffodils out and I thought about my lovely old Nan (Joaney's Mum, we were very close and I really miss her). She loved anything yellow and spring was her favourite time of year. I sat in the sun reading for a while before swimming. Found myself also reading all the dedications on the benches and feeling glad to be alive on such a lovely day and grateful for living in such a nice place.

How do I feel a year since the first chemotherapy and six months post-surgery?

+ My hair is now growing a bit thicker and is about 2cm long but it's very grey.
+ My nails still aren't growing normally so I have to keep them cut very short.
+ My eyebrows are very grey and patchy so I have to pencil them in daily.
+ My eyelashes are very short and don't seem to be growing any more.
+ My joints ache, particularly my knees and hips.
+ My left arm is still slightly swollen at the top and around my elbow, so I wear the compression sleeve for part of every day.
+ My fingertips are still numb but I'm getting fewer pins and needles in my hand.
+ My new breast is brill to look at but it still feels a bit weird having muscle in there as it feels like it could burst when I sneeze!
+ I don't like the deformity in my armpit from the lymph node dissection but find wearing vest tops under shirts and tops helps to disguise it.
+ The sensation is returning to normal slowly around the top of my arm and back area but I still can't feel when I spray deodorant in my left axilla.
+ My weight is still an issue but I can't blame fluid retention any more so will just have to eat less and move more!!
+ The Herceptin® gives me cold symptoms (cough, runny nose

and watery eyes) every three weeks and seems to make me more tired each time.

✦ I still feel tired after exercise but can do a lot more than a few months ago.

✦ I hate the menopausal symptoms but take comfort in the hope of them not lasting forever and knowing I can try different medication to help alleviate the night sweats, etc.

✦ I would love to sleep through the night without waking up at all but I can relax about it while still off work. I'm worried about how I'll cope with lack of sleep and getting up for work though.

✦ I feel calmer about my future. I still think that breast cancer may ultimately shorten my life, but I'm determined it's not going to spoil it.

✦ I've spent a fortune on vests and camisoles, books and magazines, meals out, sandwiches and cappuccinos, toiletries and make-up, new bras of various sizes and flowers but they've all helped to keep me happy!

✦ I can laugh now about the number of times I complained about taste changes during the chemo. It didn't stop me eating though and I think I've spent more this year on food and drink than ever before!

ANOTHER PROBLEM PRE-SURGERY AND THE OPERATION IS CANCELLED AGAIN

26 MARCH 2007

Really uncomfortable overnight. My breast is tight and sore when I touch it or move my arm. Decided to go to aqua aerobics and have a swim to see if it wore off. Couldn't do the arm exercises and it hurt when I ran in the water and I couldn't swim. Looks a bit pinker than the other side and the skin feels warmer.

27 MARCH 2007

Rang Eileen at BUPA as I've still got pain and the tightness. Phil Turton is away but she thought I ought to see someone so went in to see another surgeon. He thought that, as the skin was tense, pinker and warmer, I should have some antibiotics and see Phil

Turton pre-op on Monday. Started flucloxacillin and will possibly need antibiotic cover post-op too. I just hope it won't stop things happening next Wednesday as I've just got the letter for admission and have to be in at 3pm.

Eileen said I'll have to go to St James's for the guidewire to be inserted for removing the calcification and I guess that will be in the morning, so not really looking forward to 4th April.

As I can't swim with the inflammation I decided to go for a walk in the afternoon and sat in the churchyard reading. By chance I saw the memorial stone of a nurse I knew from Cookridge who died at the age of 58 years. Felt sad for her as there were no flowers from anyone. I keep thinking about death, but then I always have done and I don't think I'm getting more morbid generally.

31 MARCH 2007

Feel a bit despondent today as I've nearly finished the flucloxacillin and my breast is still swollen and pink. Went over to my parents and took them out for lunch. I'm beginning to think the surgery will be cancelled again.

1 APRIL 2007

Not a good day for my family, Steve rang and both my parents in hospital – Joaney with her heart problem and Pop fell at home, so Steve had to take him to A&E as he hurt his hand and cut his head.

2 APRIL 2007

Rang the hospitals about my parents and then went into work to meet Janet Brown, the new consultant I'll be working with in the renal cancer clinic. Caught up with a few people and it was good to see them.

Saw Phil Turton and he wants me to have high dose flucloxacillin and ciprofloxacin for two weeks. He thinks the implant might be infected and may need to be removed. He reassured me that 90% of the tissue is my own so not having the implant shouldn't make too much difference to the breast shape. He just needed to add it at the time of surgery to give a fuller shape. I can't go ahead with the other surgery until this is sorted out and it could be a few weeks or months. He doesn't want me to work until the inflammation is sorted and so I've no choice but to be patient.

Pop back at home today after having hourly neurological obs all night. He was dropped off at lunchtime by ambulance and it's a worry that he's on his own.

5 APRIL 2007

Joaney home today, but has caught a bug from the ward so is feeling awful. She's told me to stay away as she doesn't want to pass it on.

9 APRIL 2007

Easter Monday. Went to see Joaney and Pop. They both look frail. Joaney has lost weight and is tiny now, and Pop has a huge swollen lump and bruise on his head and awful black eyes. Went to Steve's to be with the rest of the family and had a good time despite the upset and worry of our parents.

10 APRIL 2007

Herceptin® again today. Only two more to go. Eileen came to check my breast and drew round the inflamed area with a pen to monitor the area of pinkness. It's definitely improving so she rang Phil Turton and he wants to see me on the 13th as planned.

13 APRIL 2007

Saw Phil Turton again and he was pleased with the lesser area of inflammation, but wanted me to have an ultrasound to check for any possible fluid collection around the implant, which could mean there's infection around it. Luckily no fluid and the doc who did the ultrasound thought the swelling might be due to radiotherapy effects. (I later read a report on radiation fibrosis and 'capsular contraction' occurring in a high proportion of women post-skin-sparing mastectomy.)[41] So, I've to complete the antibiotics and see Phil Turton on the 20th.

I finished reading *Through A Glass, Darkly* by the philosophy writer Jostein Gaarder. I love his books and this one's about a terminally ill little girl talking to her guardian angel.[42] Makes me hope that we've all got one.

16 APRIL 2007

Steve rang early. Pop fell again last night and spent all night on the bedroom floor. Joaney called an ambulance and the GP is going later as he refused to go into hospital with the paramedics. I finished the antibiotics today and am glad as they were making me nauseated.

17 APRIL 2007

Pop had to sleep in the chair last night, so Joaney stayed downstairs too. Can't think that things are going to get better. Worried all day and then Steve rang early evening. They've taken Pop into Dewsbury Hospital again. I'm glad because at least he'll be safe in there.

20 APRIL 2007

Saw Phil Turton and we have another plan. He explained about not being able to operate on both sides at once as he thinks the distortion on the left is due to the capsular contraction pulling the muscle and squashing the implant. After our holiday in June he plans to do the mastopexy to give me uplift on the right and remove the calcification from there. For the last few nights in the bath I've been feeling a lump in there but he reassured me it was from the biopsy and nothing sinister. He seemed disappointed that the left side has changed so much, and suggested I may need another implant in there at a later stage and there's no point in constructing a nipple as the areola area is now in the wrong place.

I can accept all that, and it's perhaps a good thing that I'm available to help out my parents at this time, as it might be necessary for them to move into more suitable accommodation. I've made a decision that I'll try to get back to work in May.

MY FIRST HAIRCUT IN OVER A YEAR!

21 APRIL 2007

Went to see Cathy for a trim. Told her it wouldn't take long, but she said she might get creative! She cut the frizzy grey ends so it looks darker again and put gel on the spiky bits,but it showed up how thin it is on the top of my scalp. Still feel it looks better, and hopefully people think I've just gone for a short style and I'll blend in with the public now.

Phil went with me to pick up Joaney to go see Pop in hospital. He's still got a very bruised face and he's not very talkative. He was upset when Joaney told him she can't visit every day. I'll have to try and drive over next week but at the moment my chest and arm still ache quite a bit from driving too far. Joaney liked my hair and I haven't had short hair since I had the 'basin' cut after starting junior school. I used to get home with one of my plaits undone and a ribbon missing so Joaney got a bit fed up and chopped it short!

23 APRIL 2007

Interesting how I feel the need to justify what's happened to me. I keep searching for deep and meaningful philosophical books and I realised this today when Jehovah's Witnesses came to the door. I was just about to deliver my stock answer of 'No thanks, I'm a nurse and believe in using blood products, etc.', when I spotted a heading on the front of the 'Awake' magazine. As the lady was talking I saw the title 'Is your life predestined?' and agreed to take it to read. I've always believed in fate or correct timing, such as when I met Phil and how we were both ready to fall in love again, and being successful in job interviews, etc. My good friend Caroline, who's Scottish, told me years ago 'What's for ye will no go by ye!' Anyway I read the article. It discusses whether a greater force such as God predetermines our actions and destiny, and concludes that when good or bad events happen, they're not inevitable and we map our own futures by our decisions. I was rather surprised by that as I agree, but thought that the Witnesses may believe God plays a much more significant role in our destiny. Think I'll get back to the trashy magazines and novels after this!!

1 MAY 2007

Penultimate Herceptin® today. Picked up final sick note for work from GP surgery to return as fit from today. Herceptin® went okay but my blood pressure was raised 191/109 so Jane in the IV team suggested I check it again when I get back to work at the end of the week. Went straight home afterwards to relax and stroke my cats to help lower my BP!

2 MAY 2007

Bad day, feel sick and blood 'whooshing' in my ears all day. Really tired as well so just stayed in with my cats. So ironic as I'm due back at work tomorrow. Determined to go in, even if I feel awful, I'm not changing the plans again.

'MY NAME'S KATE, I'VE HAD BREAST CANCER AND NOW I'M BACK AT WORK'

3 MAY 2007

First day back and thankfully feel better. Felt like I'd been away a lot less than 14 months or so. Worried about getting in on time but managed that okay as Phil is always good at getting up and reminded me that my 'holiday' was over! Debbie took my blood pressure in clinic and it's down to 145/99 and I thought I'd be more stressed today. Lovely to see everyone and walked into the office as Gill and Lorna were making a 'Welcome Back Kate' banner and putting up balloons for me!

Ironically, the first post I opened was from Breast Cancer Care offering a free information pack to me stating, 'Your patient has 101 questions. We have 100s of people who can help'. It made me think about all the people that have helped me: Tim Perren, Phil Turton, Catherine and the IV team, Eileen and Jeanette and ward staff at BUPA, Belinda and others in the Breast Unit at St James's, the radiographers at Cookridge and my GP for sick notes and prescriptions, not forgetting my Phil, lovely friends and family of course.

7 MAY 2007

Bank Holiday Monday. Went into work with Phil before picking Joaney up to see Pop, who's now in a nursing home for respite care until a care package is sorted at home. He looks better but not nice seeing him in there with the other 'Zimmer' users!

He asked me about work and told him I'm a bit worried about

getting up early and into work for my normal 8am start. I have to work two full days this week.

8 MAY 2007

First full day at work for me and also Joaney's 82nd birthday today. Pop rang and sang 'Happy Birthday' over the phone to her in the morning. He's upset about not getting her a present or card.

I had a good day at work catching up with colleagues and patient administration but felt exhausted by the end of the afternoon. Joked with the nurses in clinic that have been covering for me that I'm going to resign as they seemed relieved to see me back to hand over the responsibilities of the immunotherapy patients!

9 MAY 2007

Slept better than I have for a long long time. Such a relief to have a few hours of continuous sleep instead of catnapping. Beginning to look forward to clinic on Monday next week when I'll be in contact with some of my patients again. Then I'll feel like a 'proper' nurse again.

14 MAY 2007

My first kidney cancer clinic today since being back at work and I've decided this is going to be the last entry of my journal.

Well I surprised myself and loved every minute of being back in action and seeing patients again. I felt apprehensive about how I would cope with seeing my old patients from over a year ago, but in the end it was fine. A few commented on my short hair and wondered if I'd been on a 'round the world trip' but when I said 'it had been a journey of a different kind' they seemed to understand and just hoped I was now okay. I feel like I've got my old enthusiasm back to help others and relish the chance to meet new patients and offer my support as they embark on their treatment.

MY PHIL WANTED TO CONTRIBUTE TOO: THIS IS HIS SUMMARY

I didn't let Phil read any of my journal as I was writing my thoughts and I've been a bit apprehensive about his reaction to my criticism of his response to me at times. He's only ever wanted to be there for me and I know I sometimes pushed him away. I did this both physically by denying him the chance to come to my appointments and by withdrawing from him at home when I simply felt too drained to communicate.

We've talked about this since my recovery from the drug side effects and traumas, etc. Like Phil, I believe we've had our share of emotional upheavals during our relationship and although we joke about me struggling to ever say 'sorry', I am truly sorry for not being more understanding of Phil's needs and fears throughout *my* cancer experience. He's dealt bravely with his own experience and continues to do so as he remains well and healthy but the 'threat' is always there. Now it's there for both of us and I know he's forgiven me for the times we were at odds with each other. I think we both believe 'life really is too short' to spoil it. Phil wrote this as I'd finished all the major treatment:

> How should I have responded to Kate's diagnosis? After the initial shock of her announcement about her very real fears, the feeling was 'let's get on with what has to be done'. Perhaps one would have expected that to be followed by anger – the 'why us?' reaction. However, after more than our share of life's 'downs', including my own protracted fight against the disease in the 80s and 90s, I'm beyond believing that such 'challenges' are spread evenly or fairly throughout the population – why doesn't every 40-a-day smoker get lung cancer and why do volunteer charity workers get kidnapped and murdered overseas?
>
> How do I feel now? Immense relief that two key moments went for us; the immediate impact of the change in the chemo to Taxotere® in May 2006 and the results of the histology after surgery in September last year.
>
> How about the future? After being free of cancer for 15 years, and probably as a subconscious self-defence mechanism, I find difficulty in remembering much about my own experience. In a similar vein, with Kate's recent return to work and the future prognosis being

encouraging, I have probably already consigned the traumas of the last year or so to history. It is a shame that, and contrary to the views purported to be expressed by many people in our position, I do not wake up each morning vowing to make the most out of the gift of life (to travel the world, make a parachute jump, etc.). I simply hope that we can expect a decent period of normal living before life presents its next 'challenge'

THE END OF THE 'JOURNEY'?

I've achieved my goal of getting back to work and feel guilty now about wondering why women in a support group I used to attend always said 'I've had breast cancer and now I'm back at work' when they were introducing themselves. Rather uncharitably I used to wonder why they always told us that, but now I realise how important it is to feel a useful member of society again through working. A study of cancer survivors describes how time becomes divided into a 'before' and 'after'.[43] I feel like that as not only have I undergone physical changes, but I'm very aware that a whole year has passed me by and I want to 'get back to normal', which of course includes work.

I'm probably going to carry on reading related literature as I find quite a lot of comfort in other people's experiences such as this statement from another breast cancer patient: 'Whether cancer brings an early death or not it is still possible to live a life of completeness and aliveness in the time that we have left, be it a few months or many years'.[44]

I have also maintained an interest in spinal injuries since my days as both staff nurse and sister on the spinal injuries unit at Pinderfields hospital. In Christopher Reeves' last book before he died, *Nothing is Impossible: reflections on a new life*, he writes about overcoming seemingly insurmountable hardships.[45] If he truly believed that, as a C-2 vent-dependent quadriplegic with all four limbs paralysed and needing an artificial respirator to breathe, then the slight change in my physical appearance and stamina is trivial in comparison to the huge challenges he experienced. I've also just finished reading Dame Tanni Grey Thompson's book about her life as a wheelchair athlete. She talks about us all experiencing challenges that get in the way of what we're trying to do and how they can grow until they seem too big to deal with.[46] Well I feel as though I've faced a fairly big challenge over the last 14 months or so, but thankfully it's never felt insurmountable.

As I complete this account of my personal 'cancer journey' it's not quite at the end as I have a final Herceptin® infusion at the end of May and more surgery to face in the summer. However, I feel the circle is complete as I stop thinking of myself as a patient and feel more like a nurse again. Thankfully, I feel the whole experience will enhance my nursing approach to my patients but only time will tell as long as I maintain good health and revert back to being a carer again rather than a patient.

I'll leave the last words to Ernesto, one of my lovely patients who kept in touch with me by cards and email. This was his last one, 'I am really pleased that you are back at work. It will help you a lot and the wonderful humane touch that you had with the patients before being ill will be even better now'. I sincerely hope he's right.

Postscript: 'Thanks for making me feel whole again'

<u>25 JULY 2007</u>

I wasn't going to write anymore but I feel the need to 'finish things off'. I've had a bit of a wobble emotionally after completing the Herceptin® in May as I've joined the many other patients who are concerned about treatment cycles ending. I never predicted missing the three-weekly cannulation and Herceptin® infusion, but now it's finished I miss the IV team liaison and the reassurance I felt at receiving an IV drug. Despite continuing on the letrozole, which is taken orally, my patient's brain tells me it's not as 'good', while my nurse's brain knows that this is not the case.

My surgery was completed on 29th June so I feel much more symmetrical and confident in my appearance. As I write I've still got the scars taped with flesh coloured micropore to prevent them stretching, and Phil Turton has reassured me that my repositioned nipple will be okay and won't drop off as the blood supply is viable! I sent him a card last week to say, 'Thanks for making me feel whole again'. It was a cartoon of a mermaid in a bath showing off her ample chest. I'm nowhere near as attractive, but my Phil reassures me all the time that I look fine as I am. The very good news following the surgery was that the calcified area that Phil Turton removed was benign, so I'll just need yearly mammograms from now on and follow up appointments with Tim Perren.

Sad news too as our friend Sally died and we went to her funeral last week. She was only 51 and such a talented, lovely person. I cried through the majority of the service as we were sitting very close to the family and I felt so sad for them. I could see her husband Mike looking at her photo before she became ill with the brain malignancy that cut her life short. I couldn't help thinking that if my treatment hadn't been so successful, my Phil could have been in the same awful situation as Mike is now. Perhaps that's a little melodramatic, but I know Phil's been really concerned, and at times I've reacted badly to his concern and feel guilty at the distance that caused between us. Today I love him more than ever and cherish the time we're together whether doing boring, mundane day-to-day things or time spent away on holiday, eating out and the Rhinos matches!

I'm enjoying life again, but breast cancer continues its devastating impact on women's lives around me, as my friend's mum and a friend from the health club have just been diagnosed. I've tried to help allay some of their fears by talking and listening to them and feel very grateful that I'm at the final stage of treatment and not the beginning.

As for my family, ill health continues to dominate my parent's lives. As I write this, Pop is an inpatient again after only a few days at home since his last admission and Joaney is in another hospital with cardiac problems. They now need sheltered accommodation. My niece is having a difficult pregnancy with her second baby, also requiring several hospital admissions, so my poor brother Steve is getting a bit fed up with hospital visits.

In contrast, I love being back working in the hospital environment and it's only when I get a twinge of rib pain from the radiotherapy or nerve pain from the surgery that I remember the extent of my treatment (or look in the mirror, as without make-up my eyebrows and eyelashes are still very sparse). I had my hair restyled but it's still very fine and I use loads of products to spike it up to disguise my scalp and attempt a 'funky' style. Fatigue is also a problem, as I still can't sleep through the night and feel exhausted most evenings after work. Interestingly I perked up last weekend when the wine and conversation were flowing. I had cooked a meal to repay our friends Tracie and Dean for the times they catered for us during my treatment. I've also decided that Christmas dinner is going to be 'chez Hayward' again this year. So to quote Pop's favourite saying 'all being well', our joint families will be together once more from the 80 plus-year-olds to my new great niece, and we can all look forward to a good and healthy New Year.

As I reflect on being a patient and my return to being a Clinical

Nurse Specialist, I find I have increased my tolerance of patient's concerns about the everyday aspects of living with cancer. Now I listen when patients have dietary problems and can appreciate how much this affects their enjoyment of life (remember chocolate, chips and curry!). I also find I'm a bit more tolerant of medical inaccuracies with books or articles I read now, as I can appreciate the person's perception of the treatment or consultation might have led them to describe their experience inaccurately. For example, I've just finished reading a novel about breast cancer by Janice Russell who had breast cancer herself. She describes the main character as suffering bruises post-op from 'the great needle' used to deliver subcutaneous heparin.[47] At one time I would have been irritated by this line, as the needles are so small, but I can now allow for this, as the author probably had them herself and in her eyes perhaps the needle did seem huge. Indeed I've probably made mistakes in some of the descriptions of my own treatment but if so, it's because I had my 'patient head' on at the time and not my 'nurse's' one.

Similarly, Michael Gearin-Tosh referenced some of the medical staff I know in his book about rejecting conventional multiple myeloma treatment. At first I found myself wanting to defend them, particularly Prof Peter Selby, whom he accuses of not developing his point of detecting a 'morbid glamour' in reactions to cancer.[48] I read Peter's book many years ago and found it again to check up on this argument. In fact, Peter clearly defines to me that cancer is often presented with morbid glamour, as a scourge which we have brought on ourselves or that is thrust upon us uninvited.[49] However, as I continued to read Gearin-Tosh's account of his reasoning, I realised everyone has a right to interpret their cancer 'journey' as they travel through it in their own way. Inevitably, along with the gratitude for successful treatment approaches, many people need to voice their doubts and criticisms of cancer care and I hope I'll be more receptive to their concerns in the future as I continue to care for my own group of cancer patients. In the normal sense of the word, there's not much 'glamour' about having cancer, as it strips you bare both physically and mentally. Everyone desperately wants to resume a 'normal' life but I think it changes you in such a way that 'normal' is a mystery. There are days when I want to buy treats (handbags, clothes, jewellery, ice-cream, etc!) just because I'm still alive, and others when I crave forgetting about it all and pretending it never happened. Is this what being normal is?

What's the point of it all? This is a question that John Diamond's editor posed to him during his terminal illness, and I like his philosophy which was: 'It's about loving and being loved, about doing the right thing, about one day being missed when we're gone.'[50]

I'll settle for that . . .

References

1 Keswick Jencks M. *A View from the Front Line & Excerpts from a Blueprint and Constitution for a Cancer Caring Centre.* London: Expedite Graphic; 1995, p. 13.

2 Hayward K. A difficult journey through biological therapy. *Nurse2Nurse.* 2004; **3**(12): 31–3.

3 Rogers J. Follow my leader. *Cancer Nursing Practice.* 2005; **4**(8): 16–19.

4 Hayward K. Biological therapy (immunotherapy) for cancer: action and effects. *Nurse2Nurse.* 2004; **4**(6): 28–31.

5 Fentiman IS, Hamed H. *Atlas of Breast Examination.* London: BMJ Publishing Group; 1997, p. 3.

6 Fentiman IS, Hamed H. *Atlas of Breast Examination.* London: BMJ Publishing Group; 1997, p. 4.

7 Hunniford G. *Next to You: Caron's courage remembered by her mother.* London: Penguin; 2005.

8 Baum M, Saunders C, Meredith S. *Breast Cancer: a guide for every woman.* New York: Oxford University Press; 1994, pp. 5, 21.

9 Sandall R. Lost in the cancer maze. *The Sunday Times Magazine.* 10/12/2006, pp. 52–63.

10 Clark B. A life in the day. *The Sunday Times Magazine.* 18/2/2006, p. 66.

11 Cancer Research UK. *Statistics on the risk of developing cancer.* London: Cancer Research UK; January 2006.

12 Granet R. *Surviving Cancer Emotionally: learning how to heal.* New York: Wiley & Sons; 2001, p. 51.

13 Cancerbackup. *G-CSF information sheet.* London: Cancerbackup; March 2007.

14 Woodcock J. An oncological perspective. In: Salter M, editor. *Altered Body Image: the nurse's role.* 2nd edn. London: Baillière Tindall Publishing; 1997, p. 137.

15 Roche. *Breast Cancer and HER2 Testing.* Welwyn Garden City: Roche; 2005.

16 Cancerbackup. *EC chemotherapy information sheet.* London: Cancerbackup; February 2006.

17 Malo JW. *Ovulation induction drugs risk of ovarian cancer.* Available at: www.IVF.com

18 Picardie J. Can IVF cause breast cancer? *Daily Mail.* 30/09/2003.

19 Breast Cancer Care. *Factsheets: Taxotere (docetaxel).* No. 23, August 2000.

20 Oral thrush (August 19, 2005). www.mayoclinic.com/health/oral-thrush/DS00408

21 Brewer S. *The Essential Guide to Vitamins, Minerals and Supplements.* London: Market Vision Limited; 2003, p. 39.

22 Diamond J. *Because Cowards Get Cancer Too.* London: Vermilion; 1998.

23 Rosenberg SA, Barry JM. *The Transformed Cell: unlocking the mysteries of cancer.* London: Chapmans; 1993, p. 208.

24 Kintzel PE, Michaud LB, Lange MK. Docetaxel-associated epiphora. *Pharmacotherapy.* 2006; **26**(6): 853–67.

25 Cancerbackup. *Understanding Breast Reconstruction.* 8th edn. London: Cancerbackup; 2003.

26 Groopman J. *The Anatomy of Hope: how people find strength in the face of illness.* London: Simon & Schuster UK Ltd; 2005.

27 Plato. *The Republic.* Penguin Classics. Rev 2nd rp edn. London: Penguin; 1955, p. 106.

28 Hill A. Financial threat to CNSs. *Cancer Nursing Practice.* 2006; **5**(7): 12.

29 Clark B, Sitzia J, Harlow W. Incidence and risk of arm oedema following treatment for breast cancer: a three-year follow-up study. *QJM: An International Journal of Medicine.* 2005; **98**(5): 343–8.

30 Cunnick GH, Mokbel K. Oncological considerations of skin-sparing mastectomy. *International Seminars in Surgical Oncology.* **3**: 14. www.issoonline.com/content3/1/14

31 Pountney D. New gold standard. *Cancer Nursing Practice.* 2006; **5**(9): 14–16.

32 Stebbings C. How we moved on from grief. *Psychologies.* 2007; **January**: 84–7.

33 Pease A, Pease B. *Why Men Don't Have a Clue and Women Always Need More Shoes.* London: Orion; 2006.

34 Tomlinson C. Cancer's casualties: sex and love. *Cancer Nursing Practice.* 2007; **6**(2): 6–7.

35 Clark R. *A Long Walk Home.* Oxford: Radcliffe Publishing; 2002, p. 74.

36 Granet R. *Surviving Cancer Emotionally: learning how to heal.* New York: Wiley & Sons; 2001, p. 72.

37 Picardie J. *If the Spirit Moves You: life and love after death*. London: Picador; 2002.

38 Picardie J. A curl's best friend. *The Telegraph Stella Magazine*. 25/2/2007, p. 38.

39 Removing both breasts reduces cancer risk. *Journal of Clinical Oncology*. 2001; October 1. www.breastcancer.org/research_genetics_100101.html

40 Heizisouer KJ. Contralateral prophylactic mastectomy: quantifying benefits and weighing the harms. *Journal of Clinical Oncology*. 2005; **23**(19): 4251–3.

41 Mokbel R, Mokbel M. Skin-sparing mastectomy and radiotherapy: update. *International Seminars in Surgical Oncology*. 2006; **3**(35). www.issoonline.com/content/3/1/35

42 Gaarder J. *Through A Glass, Darkly*. London: Phoenix; 1999.

43 Rasmussen DM, Elverdam B. Cancer survivors' experience of time: time disruption and time appropriation. *Journal of Advanced Nursing*. 2006; **57**(6): 614–22.

44 Smith M. *Hope on the Heavy Road: learning to live with cancer*. Darlington: Scarsdale Books; 1996.

45 Reeve C. *Nothing is Impossible: reflections on a new life*. London: Century; 2002.

46 Grey Thompson T. *Aim High*. Bedlinog: Accent Press Ltd; 2007.

47 Russell J. *Keeping Abreast*. York: Insight Press; 1998, p. 78.

48 Gearin-Tosh M. *Living Proof: a medical mutiny*. London: Scribner; 2003, p. 20.

49 Wheeler S, Selby P. *Confronting Cancer Cause and Prevention*. London: Penguin; 1993, p. 3.

50 Diamond J. *Snake Oil and Other Preoccupations*. London: Vintage Publishing; 2001, p. 270.

Glossary

Alopecia: this is the term for hair loss which may be total or partial when certain chemotherapy drugs are given and also when radiotherapy is given to the brain.

Aromatase inhibitors act by blocking conversion of androgens into oestrogen in the tissues other than the ovaries. They can only be used in post-menopausal women. Letrozole is a non-steroidal aromatase inhibitor.

Axilla: medical term for the armpit.

Bendrofluazide: a diuretic drug which can help to decrease the amount of excess fluid in the body caused by some of the chemotherapy drugs.

Biological therapy: drugs that act on the bodies immune system to fight cancer cells.

Bone-density scan: a scan to measure bone strength in women at risk of osteoporosis.

Bone marrow autotransplant: for people with diseases requiring high-dose drug treatment and replacement bone marrow who haven't got a matched sibling. It's possible to take their own bone marrow before the drugs are given and then transplant it back via an intravenous drip.

Calcification: an area of white specks that show on mammography and ultrasound. A speck can be removed by biopsy to test if it is benign (non-cancerous) or malignant (cancerous).

Canesten®: an anti-fungal cream used for fungal skin infections.

Capsular contraction: after radiotherapy the area treated can tighten and if this happens after breast reconstruction the new breast shape can alter. If an implant is used also, this can be squashed and become misshapen. May need further surgery to release the hardened tissue.

Cerebrovascular accidents are commonly known as 'strokes'. They can occur in people who have hypertension (high blood pressure).

Chest x-ray: invisible rays that penetrate the area requested. Chest x-rays show the ribs, lungs and heart size.

Co-danthramer: a laxative in medicine form.

Co-dydramol: a painkiller which contains paracetamol and another drug, dihydrocodeine.

Compression sleeve: an elasticated sleeve which usually fits from the hand up to the shoulder to compress excess fluid caused by lymphoedema.

Contralateral mastectomy: some women who need a mastectomy also have the other breast removed to prevent them worrying about breast disease in the other side. This is referred to as the contralateral breast so if removed they've had a contralateral mastectomy as well.

Cyclizine: an anti-sickness drug.

Cystitis: inflammation or infection of the bladder, causes burning and stinging sensation and difficulty in passing urine. Some cytotoxic chemotherapy drugs cause bladder irritation and so patients need to drink lots of fluids to prevent this.

Cytotoxic chemotherapy: drugs that aim to destroy cancer cells but can also be toxic to normal cells such as hair, skin, etc.

DCIS: ductal carcinoma in situ, cancer cells present in the milk ducts of the breast. Can be removed by surgery.

Dexamethasone: a steroid drug used to suppress a potential allergic reaction to some of the cytotoxic chemotherapy drugs. (Also can be used to treat brain metastasis and to boost patient's appetite.)

Dysmennorrhoea: pain experienced during women's menstrual periods.

Epirubicin extravasating: epirubicin is a chemotherapy drug which is injected into a vein through an intravenous drip. If any of the drug leaks out of the vein into surrounding tissues then this is called 'extravasation'. This can cause a chemical burn to the area, so the nurses always take great care when they inject epirubicin and other similar drugs which are called 'vesicants'.

Evidence-based practice: all health professionals now work with research evidence when planning a patient's care. A lot of knowledge has been gained through clinical drug trials which now inform current practice.

Flotron: a machine used to help eliminate excess fluid in the legs and used post-operatively to aid circulation whilst bed-ridden. It consists of a pump which blows air to inflate and deflate plastic cuffs from ankle to calf and so the circulation is boosted while the patient is immobile.

G-CSF: granulocyte-colony stimulating factor given by injection under the skin to boost the total white blood cell count.

Granulocytes are a type of white blood cell that when looked at under the microscope have 'granules' in them.

Granisetron: an anti-sickness drug to prevent nausea and vomiting induced by some cytotoxic chemotherapy drugs.

Herceptin®: a drug given as an infusion by intravenous drip. Used in breast cancer care for women who are HER-2 positive which means they overexpress the human epidermal growth factor receptor 2 which can cause tumour growth. Herceptin® can switch off this response. When given with some other drugs it can cause heart problems. Women have regular ultrasound scans of the heart to check it's functioning normally. In some cases the years treatment may have to be stopped sooner.

Isotope injection: a radioactive substance that is given a few hours before a bone scan so the bone structure can clearly be seen on screen. It's potentially dangerous to unborn children so shouldn't mix with pregnant women during this time.

Latissimus dorsi reconstruction: a type of breast reconstruction which specialised breast surgeons perform using the patient's latissimus dorsi muscle from their back and transferring it round to the front to form a breast shape. Sometimes need to use an implant as well to improve the overall shape.

Letrozole: a hormone antagonist which works against the hormone oestrogen. Oestrogen can encourage tumour growth in women whose breast cancer is hormone-receptor positive.

Lignocaine gel: is a local anaesthetic drug in gel form which acts at the skin surface level to help with painful conditions as it numbs the area.

Lymphoedema: accumulation of lymph fluid which can arise from removal of the lymph nodes and the fluid then can cause swelling in a limb.

Lymphoma and Hodgkin lymphoma: cancer of the lymphoid tissue in the body. Can be either in the lymph nodes or lymphatic cells in organs. Hodgkin lymphoma is recognised in the laboratory because a biopsy sample has specific cells present.

Malignant melanoma: a type of skin cancer that is usually associated with sunburn and prolonged sun exposure.

Mastopexy: the name for surgery which lifts the breast tissue and repositions the nipple. Often needed to make the chest area more equal after breast cancer surgery.

Maxolon®: an anti-sickness drug which can help stop feelings of nausea and prevent vomiting.

Movicol®: a laxative in powder form which has to be mixed with water before drinking.

Multidisciplinary team (MDT) meeting: this involves cancer care health professionals from medicine, nursing, radiology, research, pathology, palliative care, etc. The patients are discussed to utilise the gathered expertise to form their treatment plan and ensure a correct diagnosis.

Myocardial infarction: a type of 'heart attack'. This causes the heart muscle to be damaged as there is lack of blood supply to it, usually from narrowing of the arteries.

Nadir: in cancer care relates to the time post-chemotherapy when the blood counts will be at their lowest point.

Neulasta growth factors: a type of G-CSF injection which boosts the total white blood cell count to prevent infections post-chemotherapy.

Neutropenia/neutropenic: these terms are used when the neutrophil count is low in the total white cell count. Neutropenia is a decrease in the neutrophil level and the patient is then described as being neutropenic.

Neutrophils: one type of white blood cell that needs to be checked regularly post-chemotherapy.

Nodal spread: cancer cells which have spread into the lymph nodes in the armpit from the breast area.

Nurse-led service: some cancer patients can be seen by nurses rather than doctors in the clinic area before continuing their treatment with chemotherapy or biological therapy. This often speeds up the process for the patient as they see the same nurse who can support the patient and family through their treatment plan.

Nystatin suspension: a liquid drug which has a dropper included to measure the correct amount prescribed to put in the mouth for oral thrush (candidiasis).

Oedematous: term used for oedema (excess fluid), in certain parts of the body such as face, legs, etc., i.e. 'my legs were oedematous'.

Osteoporosis: thinning of the bones which can lead to fractures if not treated. Post-menopausal women are at risk because of lack of oestrogen which helps normal bone growth.

PCAS: patient controlled analgesia system which is attached to a drip containing pain killers. The patient has control of a button which allows them to boost the amount of painkilling drug that flows in the drip themselves.

Peau d'orange skin: the name for skin that is pitted just like orange-peel.

Placebo effect: this is a term used for when the patient feels better because they think they are receiving an effective treatment. This is common in complementary medicine and placebo drugs are used in clinical trials to test whether the actual drug has a true effect on the disease process.

Prophylactic mastectomy: women with a very strong family history and personal risk of developing breast cancer, may choose to have their healthy breasts removed to prevent it.

Prophylactic oral antibiotics: used in cancer care when the white blood cells are low to act against any potential infections which the patient might be at risk from post-chemotherapy.

Radiation fibrosis: a rare condition post-radiotherapy when the lung tissue can become stiff and fibrous causing cough and breathlessness.

Renal cell carcinoma: a type of kidney cancer which can be treated by surgery and biological therapy.

Self-lymphatic drainage: a technique which can be done by the patient to massage specific areas of their body to aid lymph fluid drainage and help decrease tissue swelling.

Seroma: build-up of fluid under the skin causing swelling after surgery most often around the operation scar.

Stereotactic-guided core biopsy: removal of a sample of tissue to be checked in the laboratory for cancer type using x-rays and a mammogram machine to identify the suspicious area on screen.

Supraclavicular fossa: name for the area just above the collar bone.

Temozolamide: a cytotoxic chemotherapy drug used to treat malignant brain tumours called gliomas.

Tetracycline: an antibiotic that is effective for spotty skin infections which can be side effects of other drugs.

Tramadol: a painkiller used for moderate to severe pain.

Ultrasound-guided biopsy: removal of a sample of tissue to be checked in the laboratory for cancer type using ultrasound waves to identify the suspicious area on screen.

Urological: relates to the bladder, ureters (tubes from the kidneys), etc.

Venlafaxine: an antidepressant which can be used to treat hot flushes in post-menopausal women.

White count: the white cells in the blood that need to be at a high enough level to prevent patients getting infections post-chemotherapy.